Pediatric Drug Dosages

Pediatric Drug Dosages

Sunil Natha Mhaske MBBS, MD
Pediatrician and Neonatologist
Professor and Head
Department of Pediatrics
and Vice-Principal (PG)
Mail: sunilmhaske1970@gmail.com

Mitesh Chawda MBBS, DCH
Department of Pediatrics

Liza Bulsara MBBS, MD (Pediatrics)
Department of Pediatrics

Thaslima Kalathingal MBBS, MD (Pediatrics)
Department of Pediatrics

Dr Vithalrao Vikhe Patil Foundation's Medical College
Ahmednagar, Maharashtra

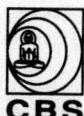

CBS

CBS Publishers & Distributors Pvt Ltd

New Delhi • Bengaluru • Chennai • Kochi • Kolkata • Mumbai

Bhopal • Bhubaneswar • Hyderabad • Jharkhand • Nagpur • Patna • Pune • Uttarakhand • Dhaka (Bangladesh)

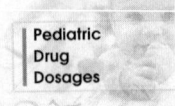

Pediatric
Drug
Dosages

ISBN: 978-93-86310-69-9

Copyright © Authors and Publisher

First Edition: 2017

Reprint: 2019

Published by Satish Kumar Jain and Produced by Varun Jain for

CBS Publishers & Distributors Pvt Ltd
4819/XI Prahlad Street, 24 Ansari Road, Daryaganj, New Delhi 110 002, India
Ph: 23289259, 23266861, 23266867   Fax: 011-23243014   Website: www.cbspd.com
e-mail: delhi@cbspd.com; cbspubs@airtelmail.in.

Corporate Office: 204 FIE, Industrial Area, Patparganj, Delhi 110 092
Ph: 4934 4934   Fax: 4934 4935   e-mail: publishing@cbspd.com; publicity@cbspd.com

Branches

- **Bengaluru:** Seema House 2975, 17th Cross, K.R. Road,
  Banasankari 2nd Stage, Bengaluru 560 070, Karnataka
  Ph: +91-80-26771678/79   Fax: +91-80-26771680   e-mail: bangalore@cbspd.com
- **Chennai:** 7, Subbaraya Street, Shenoy Nagar, Chennai 600 030, Tamil Nadu
  Ph: +91-44-26680620, 26681266   Fax: +91-44-42032115   e-mail: chennai@cbspd.com
- **Kochi:** 42/1325, 1326, Power House Road, Opp. KSEB Power House
  Ernakulam 682 018, Kochi, Kerala
  Ph: +91-484-4059061-65   Fax: +91-484-4059065   e-mail: kochi@cbspd.com
- **Kolkata:** 6/B, Ground Floor, Rameswar Shaw Road, Kolkata 700 014, West Bengal
  Ph: +91-33-22891126, 22891127, 22891128   e-mail: kolkata@cbspd.com
- **Mumbai:** 83-C, Dr E Moses Road, Worli, Mumbai 400018, Maharashtra
  Ph: +91-22-24902340/41   Fax: +91-22-24902342   e-mail: mumbai@cbspd.com

Representatives

• **Bhopal**	0-8319310552	• **Bhubaneswar** 0-9911037372	• **Hyderabad** 0-9885175004
• **Jharkhand**	0-9811541605	• **Nagpur** 0-9421945513	• **Patna** 0-9334159340
• **Pune**	0-9623451994	• **Uttarakhand** 0-9716462459	• **Dhaka (Bangladesh)** 01912-003485

Printed at Rashtriya Printers, Dilshad Garden, Delhi, India

Preface

I am very pleased to have an opportunity to pen *Pediatric Drug Dosages*. This book is designed for complete practical guidelines of dosing and usage of medication in children. Pediatric doses are a complex topic in clinical practice as it changes with age, weight, surface area and disease. Overdosing may lead to side effects and toxicity. Underdosing is not beneficial or leads to resistance to antibiotics. This book is possible due to ever gracious blessings of Almighty and my parents. Special thanks to Dr Sujay Vikhe Patil (CEO), Lt Gen (Retd) Dr B Sadananda (Secretary General), Dr Abhijit Diwate (Deputy Director), Air Mshl (Retd) Dr Dhananjay Joshi (Principal), Lt Col (Retd) Dr AK Pandey (Medical Superintendent), Dr RB Kothari (Associate Prof), my residents Dr Liza, Dr Aditya, Dr Kanchan, Dr Ninza, Dr Amit, Dr Bipin, Dr Thaslima, and with undeniable support of my beloved wife Dr Rekha Mhaske, my kids Ruchaa and Prabhat.

For any suggestion or improvement, please contact me at sunilmhaske1970@gmail.com.

Sunil Natha Mhaske

Contents

Pediatric Drug Therapy

Pharmacology: Greek word *pharmakon* means "poison" in classic Greek; "drug" in modern Greek.

The branch of medicine and biology concerned with the study of drug action is known as pharmacology.

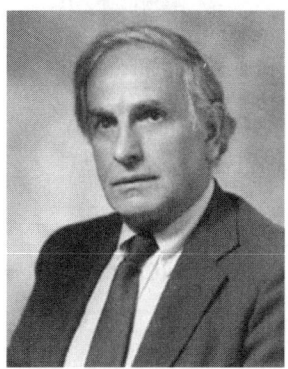

Sumner J Yaffe
Father of Pediatric Clinical
Pharmacology

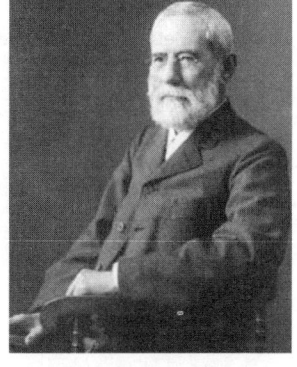

Oswald Schmiedeberg
Father of Modern
Pharmacology

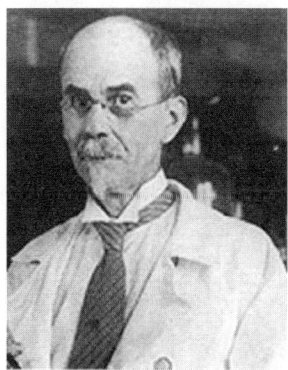

John Jacob Abel
Father of American
Pharmacology

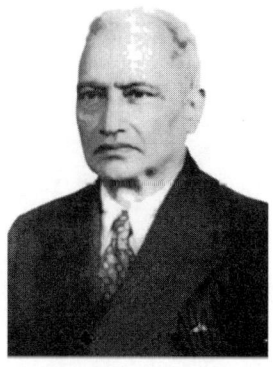

Ram Nath Chopra
Father of Indian
Pharmacology

Pharmacokinetics

Routes of Drug Administration

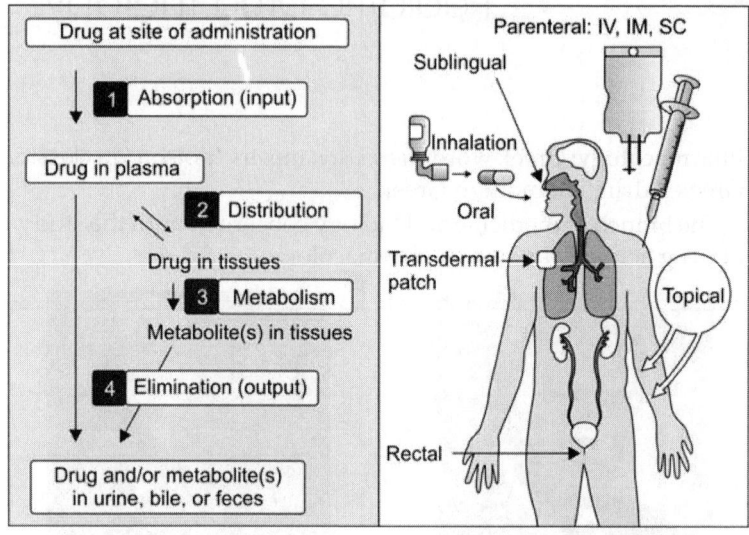

(*Courtesy:* Internet)

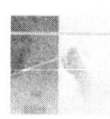

Prescription Abbreviations

WEIGHT AND MEASURES

cc	Cubic centimeter
g	Gram
kg	Kilogram
m²	Meter square
mg	Milligram
µg	Microgram
ml	Millilitre
ng	nanogram

LATIN ABBREVIATIONS AND THEIR MEANINGS

ac (ante cibum)	Before meals
Aq (aqua)	Water
bid (bis in die)	Twice a day
hs (hora sommi)	At bedtime
Liq	A liquor
Mist (mistura)	A mixture
Omn Hor (omni hora)	Every hour
Omn Man (omni mane)	Every morning
pc (post cibum)	After meals
prn (pro re nata)	As occasion arises
q (quaque)	Every
qid (quarter in die)	Four times a day
qs (quantum sufficient)	A sufficient quantity
Rx	Take (thou) a recipe
sos (siopus sit)	As and when requires
Stat (statim)	Immediately
tid (ter in die)	Three times a day

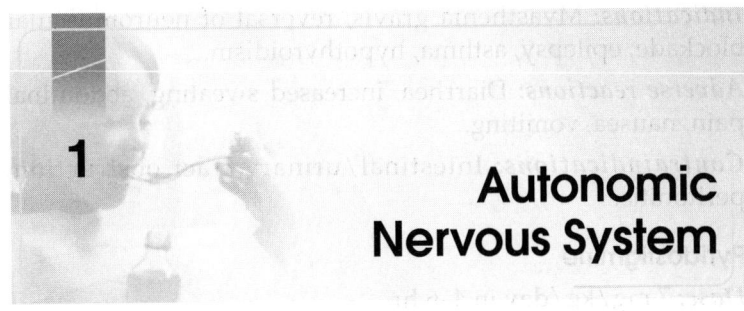

1 Autonomic Nervous System

Pilocarpine

Adult dose: 2–4 mg PO

Indication: Atropine toxicity

Adverse reactions: Sweating, salivation, tachycardia, meiosis.

Physostigmine

Dose: 0.02 mg/kg/dose IM/IV

OR 0.5 mg IV/SC/IM every 5 min

Maximum dose: 2 mg

Indications: Dhatura poisoning, atropine toxicity, open angle glaucoma.

Adverse reactions: Bradycardia, asystole, seizure, meiosis, increased muscle tone.

Contraindications: Glaucoma, asthma.

Neostigmine

Dose:

Neonate: 1 mg q4 hr, 30 min before feed

Children: 1–3 mg/kg/day oral q4–6 hr

- Begin with lower dose and increase gradually till symptoms disappear.
- Use with atropine for nondepolarising neuromuscular blocking agents.

Indications: Myasthenia gravis, reversal of neuromuscular blockade, epilepsy, asthma, hypothyroidism.

Adverse reactions: Diarrhea, increased sweating, abdominal pain, nausea, vomiting.

Contraindications: Intestinal/urinary tract obstruction, peritonitis.

Pyridostigmine

Dose: 7 mg/kg/day in 4–6 hr

Indication: Myasthenia gravis

Contraindication: Epilepsy

Adverse reactions: Bradycardia, headache, salivation, meiosis.

Edrophonium

Dose:

Initial dose: 0.04 mg/kg/dose

Maximum dose: 1 mg for <30 kg

If no response after 1 min, may give 0.16 mg/kg/dose for total of 0.2 mg/kg.

Maximum dose: 5 mg for <30 kg

Indication: For diagnosis of myasthenia gravis

Contraindication: Epilepsy

Adverse reactions: Arrhythmias, hypotension, drowsiness.

Atropine

Dose: Preanaesthesia: IV/IM; For <5 kg weight 0.04 mg/kg dose.

For >5 kg weight: 0.03 mg/kg/dose

Sinus bradycardia: IV 0.02 mg/kg

Organophosphate poisoning: 0.05 mg/kg IV repeat every 5–10 minutes till secretions are dried.

Once atropinization is achieved repeat doses every 30–60 minutes or give IV infusion 0.02–0.08 mg/kg/hr

Bronchospasm: Inhalation 0.03–0.05 mg/kg/dose 3–4 times/day.

Indications: Antidote of choice for both organophosphate and carbamate poisoning, preanaesthesia, sinus bradycardia, heart block.

Contraindications: Thyrotoxicosis, GI-tract disease uropathy.

Adverse reaction: Tachycardia

Hyoscine Butylbromide

Dose:

- 6–12 years: oral: 10 mg q6 hr
- IV/IM: 10–20 mg bolus

Indications: Motion sickness prophylaxis, intestinal and biliary colic.

Contraindications: Megacolon, glaucoma.

Adverse reactions: Tachycardia, sedation, anticholinergic side effects.

Ipratropium

Dose: Neonates: 25 µg/kg/dose 3 times/day as nebulisation

Children: 125–250 µg as nebulisation

Indications: Acute and chronic asthma, COPD

Adverse reactions: Tachycardia, drowsiness, xerostomia, blurred vision.

Glycopyrrolate

Dose: PO: 40–100 µg/kg/dose 3–4 times/day

Indication: Used as a preanaesthetic medication to decrease secretions and reflex bronchospasm during GA.

Contraindication: Down syndrome

Adverse reactions: Brain damage, spastic paralysis

Dicyclomine

Dose:

- 6 months–2years: 10–20 drops 15 minutes before feed
- >2 years: 1 ml every 6 hr

Adult dose: 10–20 mg TDS

Indications: Treatment of urinary incontinence, functional disturbances of GI motility

Contraindications: GI obstruction, urinary tract obstruction

Adverse reactions: Tachycardia, spastic paralysis.

Adrenaline

Dose:

- For IV/*intraosseous use for cardiac arrest:* 0.1 ml/kg/dose of 1: 10,000 solution
- For *endotracheal use:* 0.1 mg/kg/dose of 1: 1000 solution
- For *nonresponse during CPR:* 0.1 ml/kg of 1: 10000 solution IV repeated every 3–5 minutes
- *Anaphylaxis and bronchial asthma:* 0.01 ml/kg (1:1000 solution) IM, can be repeated at 15–30 minutes interval.
- For *shock:* 0.1–1 µg/kg/min IV

Indications: DOC for anaphylactic shock, cardiac arrest, bronchospasm, anaphylactic reaction.

Adverse reactions: Pallor, tachycardia, headache, tremor.

- 1: 1000 solution means 1 ml = 1 mg
- 1: 10,000 solution means 1 ml = 0.1 mg

Noradrenaline

Dose: 0.05–0.1 µg/kg/min

Indications: Shock, hypotension

Adverse reactions: Arrhythmia, bradycardia, tachycardia, organ ischemia.

Dopamine

Dose: 1–20 µg/kg/minute

Indications: Drug of choice for cardiogenic shock with oliguric renal failure, hypotension

Adverse reactions: Decreased urine output, tachycardia, arrhythmia.

Ephedrine

Dose: 2 drops in each nostril 2–3 times a day

Indication: Nasal congestion.

Phenylephrine

Dose:
- 1–2 drops/nostril q6h (nasal congestion)
- 1 drop 15–30 min, before procedure (ophthalmic procedure)

Indication: Nasal congestion, as mydriatic in ophthalmic procedure.

Adverse reaction: Rebound congestion on prolonged nasal use.

Dobutamine

Dose: 5–20 µg/kg/min IV

Indication: Hypotension

Adverse reactions: Tachycardia, ectopics, tachyarrhythmia.

Salbutamol

Dose:

Oral: 0.1–0.4 mg/kg/dose every 8 hr

For acute exacerbation: Up to three treatments of 2–4 puffs (100 µg/puff) by metered dose inhaler at 20 min intervals followed by 2 puffs every 4–6 hr.

Nebulization: 0.15 mg/kg/dose every 20 min for 3 doses through a nebulizer using airflow of 6 L/min.

Indication: Bronchospasm in asthma

Adverse reactions: Tachycardia, palpitation, hyperglycemia, tremor, insomnia.

Salmeterol

Dose:
- 50–100 µg/day
- 1–2 puffs twice a day
- Maximum 4 puffs twice a day or rotacap once or twice a day.

Indication: Treatment of nocturnal and exercise induced asthma as an add-on therapy to inhaled steroids.

Adverse reactions: Tachycardia, headache, muscle tremor.

Contraindication: Children <4 years.

Terbutaline

Dose:
- PO: 0.1–0.15 mg/kg/dose q8 hr
- SC: 0.005–0.01 mg/kg/dose, IM, slow IV 8 hr

Nebulisation:
- For children <20 kg: 2.5 mg
- For children >20 kg: 5 mg

Inhalation: 1–2 puffs q6–8 hr of 250 µg

Indication: Asthma

Adverse reactions: Tachycardia, headache, tremor, palpitation, arrhythmia, hypertension.

Phenoxybenzamine

Dose: PO: 0.02–2.0 mg/kg/day as single dose

Indication: Treatment of sweating and hypertension in patient with pheochromocytoma.

Adverse reactions: Nasal congestion, dizziness, constricted pupil.

Prazosin

Dose:
- *As an hypertensive not recommended in children:* 2.5 mg once a day. Maximum dose: 20 mg.
- *As a vasodilator:* PO: 10–50 µg/kg/dose q6–8 hr

Maximum: 0.1 mg/kg/dose.

For scorpion sting: 0.25 mg oral 4–6 hr for 24 hr

Indications: Mild to moderate hypertension, Raynaud's disease, scorpion sting.

Contraindication: Hypersensitivity to prazosin

Adverse reactions: Postural hypotension, syncope, dizziness, nasal stuffiness, priapism.

Tolazoline

Dose: 1–2 mg/kg IV over 10 minutes loading dose, if oxygenation improves follow it up by 0.2 mg/kg/ hr IV continuous infusion.

Indication: Pulmonary arterial hypertension in newborns with respiratory distress syndrome.

Hypertensive crisis in clonidine withdrawal and cheese reaction.

Adverse reactions: Hypotension, GI bleed, thrombocytopenia, oliguria.

Phentolamine

Dose:

- *Extravasation:* Dilute 2.5–5.0 mg in 10 ml NS and then infiltrate by multiple injections.
- *Pheochromocytoma:* IV 0.05–1.0 mg/kg/dose.

Indications: Extravasation of drugs with alpha adrenergic effects, during pheochromocytoma surgery for treatment of hypertensive crisis.

Adverse reactions: Tachycardia.

Chlorpromazine

Dose: As antipsychotic, antiemetic; PO, IV, IM: 0.5–1.0 mg/kg/dose q6–8 hr

Maximum dose:

- 1–5 years: 40 mg/day
- 5–12 years: 75 mg/day

Chorea: 50 mg/day till chorea is controlled, increase by 25 mg/day. Maximum dose: 300 mg/day.

Neonatal tetanus: 1–2 mg/kg/dose 2–4 hourly.

Amphetamine toxicity: 1 mg/kg IV/IM. Maximum dose: 50 mg.

Indications: Drug of choice for intractable hiccups, chorea, agitation, antipsychotic, mania, drug induced and postoperative nausea and vomiting, neonatal tetanus.

Adverse reactions: Postural hypotension, tachycardia, weight gain, cholestatic jaundice, extrapyramidal reactions like tardive dyskinesia, dystonia, dry mouth.

Contraindications: Avoid in children <1 year, bone marrow depression, coma, severe CNS depression.

Propranolol

Dose:

Hypertension:

- PO: 0.5–1.0 mg/kg/day
- IV: 0.01–0.1 mg/kg/dose over 15 minutes.

Maximum dose:

- In infants: 1 mg
- In children: 3 mg

Prophylaxis of migraine: PO: 0.6–1.5 mg/kg/day. Maximum dose: 4 mg/kg/day.

For cyanotic spells: PO: 2–6 mg/kg/day q6–8 hr

For arrhythmias:

- PO: 0.5–1 mg/kg/day q6 hr
- IV: 0.01–0.25 mg/kg/dose repeat in 15 minutes and then q4–8 hr.

Thyrotoxicosis: PO– 2 mg/kg/day

Indications: Hypertension, essential tremors, anxiety during pheochromocytoma surgery, capillary haemangioma, migraine prophylaxis, cyanotic spells, tachyarrhythmias, thyrotoxicosis.

Contraindications: Congestive heart failure, bronchial asthma, heart block.

Adverse reactions: Bradycardia, hypotension, hypoglycaemia in diabetics, bronchospasm, cold and clammy skin.

Sotalol

Dose: 2–8 mg/kg/day q8–12 hr

Indication: Supraventricular and ventricular arrhythmias.

Labetalol

Dose:

- PO: 4 mg/kg/day 12 hrly. Maximum dose: 40 mg/kg/day.
- For hypertensive crisis-IV: Starting dose: 0.25–1 mg/kg/dose. Continuous infusion: 0.4–1 mg/kg/hour. Maximum 3 mg/kg/hr

Indications: All grades of hypertension, hypertensive emergencies, pheochromocytoma, clonidine withdrawal.

Contraindications: Bronchial asthma, congestive heart failure (CHF), hypoglycemia, cardiogenic shock, pulmonary edema.

Adverse reactions: Postural hypotension, bradycardia, headache, conduction disturbances.

Atenolol

Dose: PO: 0.5–2 mg/kg/day

Indications: Hypertension, arrhythmia, angina

Contraindications: Bronchial asthma, pulmonary edema, cardiogenic shock, heart block, CHF.

Adverse reactions: Bradycardia, constipation, cold periphery, lethargy, depression.

Metoprolol

Dose:
- PO: 1–4 mg/kg/day 12 hrly. Maximum dose: 6 mg/kg
- For cyanotic spells: 0.1 mg/kg over 1–2 minutes repeated 5–10 minutes.

Indications: Hypertension, arrhythmias, supraventricular tachycardia, migraine prophylaxis.

Contraindications: Cardiogenic shock, CHF, bronchial asthma, sick sinus syndrome, heart block.

Adverse reactions: Bradycardia, bronchospasm, tiredness, dizziness.

Acetazolamide

Dose:
- For refractory seizures and glaucoma, raised intracranial pressure: 8–30 mg/kg/day
- *Diuretic:* 5 mg/kg/day q8 hr
- *Hydrocephalus:* PO: 50–70 mg/kg/day q8 hr

Indications: Refractory seizures and glaucoma as diuretic, hydrocephalus, to alkalinize urine in UTI, acute mountain sickness.

Contraindications: Hepatic and renal insufficiency, sodium and potassium depletion.

Adverse reactions: Drowsiness, hypokalemia, hyperglycemia, metabolic acidosis, renal calculi.

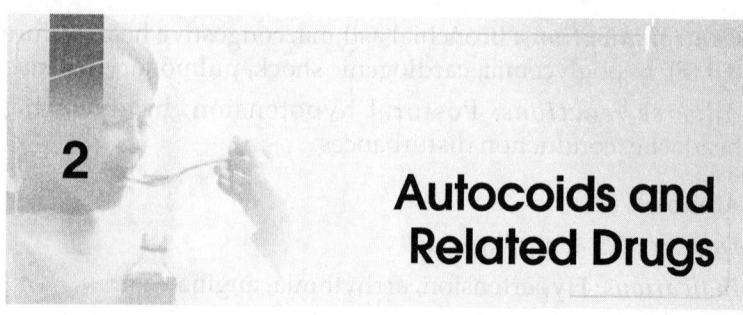

2

Autocoids and Related Drugs

HISTAMINES AND ANTIHISTAMINES

HISTAMINES

Betahistine (Vertin)

Dose: 8–16 mg thrice a day after meals.

Indications: Control of vertigo in Meniere's disease, tinnitus.

Contraindications: Avoid in <12 years of age, asthamatic and ulcer patients.

ANTIHISTAMINES

1. H1 Antagonist

A. Highly Sedative

Diphenhydramine

Dose:

- For allergic reactions/dystonia: 5 mg/kg/day q6 hr oral.
- Maximum dose: 300 mg/day.
- For anaphylaxis or phenothiazine overdose (extrapyramidal reactions): 1–2 mg/kg IV every 30 minutes repeated every 3–4 hr IM or PO.

Indications: Allergic reactions, extrapyramidal reactions, motion sickness, cough, parkinsonism, acute muscle dystonia, pruritides.

Adverse reactions: Sedation, drowsiness, psychomotor impairement, anticholinergic side effects.

Contraindications: With MAOI, bronchial asthma, porphyria, narrow angle glaucoma, urinary retention.

Dimenhydrinate

Dose: 5 mg/kg/day q6 hr oral/IM/IV.

Maximum dose:
* 2–6 years: 75 mg/day
* 6–12 years: 150 mg/day

Adult dose: 100–150 mg 8–12 hr.

Indications: Motion sickness, vertigo, radiation or cancer chemotherapy induced nausea, vomiting.

Adverse reactions: Sedation, anticholinergic. Side effects—dry mouth, urinary retention, blurring of vision.

Contraindications: Avoid in children <2 years of age, porphyria.

Promethazine

Dose:
* For nausea and vomiting: 0.25–0.5 mg/kg/dose 4–6 hr oral/ IV/IM/PR
* For motion sickness: 0.5 mg/kg/dose 12 hr oral (start half an hour before journey).
* For allergy: 0.1 mg/kg/dose
* For preoperative and postoperative sedation: 0.5–1 mg/kg/ dose.

Indications: Prophylaxis of motion sickness, chemotherapy induced vomiting, vertigo, preanaesthetic medication.

Contraindication: In children <2 years due to respiratory depression.

Adverse reactions: Drowsiness, anticholinergic side effects like dry mouth, blurring of vision, urinary retention, CNS depression.

Hydroxyzine

Dose:
* Oral: 2 mg/kg/day
* IM: 0.5–1 mg/kg/dose

Indications: As an anxiolytic, allergy, preanaesthetic medication, vomiting.

Adverse reactions: Drowsiness, hypotension, pain at injection site, dry mouth.

Contraindication: In children <1year of age, acute porphyria.

B. Moderately Sedative

Pheniramine (Avil)

Dose: 0.5 mg/kg/day oral, IM, IV

Indications: For all allergic conditions like rhinitis, conjunctivitis, urticaria, pruritis, drug allergy.

Adverse reactions: Anticholinergic side effects like dry mouth, urinary retention, sedation, blurring of vision, oculogyric spasms.

Contraindications: Epilepsy, asthma and neonates.

Cyproheptadine

Dose:
- PO: 0.25 mg/kg/day q8 hr
- 2–6 years: 2 mg/dose 8 hr (Maximum dose: 12 mg/day)
- 7–14 years: 4 mg/dose 8 hr (Maximum dose: 16 mg/day)

Indications: Loss of appetite, to promote weight gain, prophylaxis of migraine, allergic disorders.

Adverse reactions: Anticholinergic side effects like dry mouth, blurring of vision, sedation, GI upset and oculogyric spasms.

Contraindications: Urinary retention, glaucoma, hypersensitivity, asthma, neonates, with MAOI.

Meclizine

Dose:
- Motion sickness: >12 years: 2.5–25 mg oral one hour before journey.
- Vertigo: >12 years: 25–100 mg/day oral.

Indications: Motion sickness prophylaxis, vertigo.

Adverse reactions: Drowsiness, blurring of vision, dry mouth.

Contraindication: Hypersensitivity to meclizine

Cinnarizine

Dose:
- For motion sickness: 5–12 years: 12.5–25 mg 2 hr before journey.
- And 12.5 mg q8 hr during journey.
- Vestibular disorders: 25–75 mg/dose q8 hr oral in adults.

Indications: Treatment of nausea and vertigo in Meniere's disease, motion sickness, vestibular disorders.

Adverse reactions: Drowsiness, lethargy

Contraindication: Hypersensitivity to cinnarizine.

C. Mild Sedative
Chlorpheniramine

Dose:
- 0.35 mg/kg/day oral q4–6 hr
- 1–6 years: 1 mg q4–6 hr
- 6–12 years: 2 mg q4–6 hr
- >12 years: 4 mg q4–6 hr

Indications: Drug rash, allergic conditions like rhinitis, urticaria and contact dermatitis, insect bite, motion sickness.

Adverse reactions: Drowsiness, anticholinergic side effects.

Contraindication: Hypersensitivity.

Clemastine

Dose:
- 1–3 years: 0.25 mg–0.5 mg BD
- 3–6 years: 0.5 mg BD
- 6–12 years: 0.5 1 mg BD
- >12 years: 1 mg BD.

Indications: Allergic rhinitis, urticaria, angioedema, contact dermatitis.

Adverse reactions: Drowsiness, nausea, excitability.

Contraindications:
- Narrow angle glaucoma, asthma.
- Avoid in less than 1 year of age.

Second Generation

Fexofenadine

Dose:
- 6 m–2 years: 15 mg BD
- 2–12 years: 30 mg BD
- >12 years: 60 mg BD or 120 mg OD.

Indications: Allergic rhinitis, allergic skin conditions (chronic idiopathic urticaria).

Adverse reactions: Drowsiness, headache

Contraindications: Renal dysfunction, hypokalemia

Loratadine

Dose:
- 2–12 years: <30 kg: 5 mg OD oral
- >30 kg: 10 mg OD oral

Indications:
- Allergic rhinitis, urticaria
- Adverse reactions: Nausea, headache

Contraindication: Below 2 years of age.

Desloratadine

Dose: PO
- 1–5 years: 1 mg OD
- 6–11 years: 2.5 mg OD
- >12 years: 5 mg OD

Indications: Allergic rhinitis, urticaria.

Cetirizine

Metabolite of hydroxyzine.

Dose: PO
- 6 m–2 years: 2.5 mg OD
- 2–6 years: 2.5 mg BD/5 mg OD
- >6 years: 5–10 mg OD
  OR 0.2 mg/kg once a day oral.

Indications: Allergic rhinitis, allergy to food, insect bites, ocular symptoms like redness, lacrimation and itching, adjunct in seasonal asthma, urticaria.

Adverse reactions: Sedation, drowsiness, confusion

Contraindications: Hypersensitivity to cetirizine, hydroxyzine.

Levocetirizine

Levoform of cetirizine. More potent and less sedative. Effective at half the dose of cetirizine.

Dose:
- 2–6 years: 0.125 mg/kg/day single dose
- >6 years: 2.5 mg oral in a single or double dose
- Avoid below 2 years of age.

Mizolastine

Dose: >12 years: 10 mg OD

Adult dose: 10 mg OD oral

Contraindications: Hypokalemia, long QT interval, significant bradycardia.

Ebastine

Dose: >6 years: 5 mg OD

Adult dose: 10–20 mg oral OD

Indication: Nasal and skin allergy

Contraindication: Cardiac arrhythmias.

2. H_2 Antagonist
A. Cimetidine

Dose: IM/IV/PO

Neonates: 5–10 mg/kg/day q6 hr

Infants: 10–20 mg/kg/day q6 hr

Children: 20–40 mg/kg/day q6 hr

Indications: Treatment and prophylaxis of duodenal and gastric ulcers, Zollinger-Ellison syndrome, gastroesophageal reflux disease, prophylaxis of aspiration pneumonia.

Adverse reactions: Headache, dizziness, bowel upset, dry mouth, rash, bolus IV infusion has caused arrhythmia, bradycardia and cardiac arrest; gynaecomastia.

B. Ranitidine

Dose:
- 2–4 mg/kg/day q12 hr oral for 4–6 weeks (maximum dose for treatment: 300 mg/day and maintenance 150 mg/day)
- IV dose is half of oral dose
- For erosive gastritis: 4–10 mg/kg/day q12 hr

Indications: Duodenal and gastric ulcer, GERD, erosive oesophagitis, gastrinoma.

Adverse reactions: Headache, diarrhea/constipation, dizziness

Contraindication: Use cautiously in liver and renal impairment.

Famotidine

Dose: PO
- 0.5 mg/kg/day at bedtime or twice a day (maximum dose: 40 mg).
- For GERD:
  - <3 months: 0.5 mg/kg/dose once daily
  - >1year: 1 mg/kg/day twice a day (maximum dose: 80 mg)

Indications: Duodenal or gastric ulcer, GERD, ZE syndrome, prevention of aspiration pneumonia.

Adverse reactions: Headache, dizziness, constipation/diarrhea.

Contraindication: Gastric malignancy.

Roxatidine

Adult dose: 150 mg at bedtime or 75 mg BD; maintenance 75 mg at bedtime.

5-HT ANTAGONIST AND ERGOT ALKALOIDS

A. 5-HT ANTAGONISTS
Cyproheptadine
- PO: 0.25 mg/kg/day q8 hr

- 2–6 years: 2 mg/dose 8 hr (maximum dose: 12 mg/day)
- 7–14 years: 4 mg/dose 8 hr (maximum dose: 16 mg/day)

Indications: Loss of appetite, to promote weight gain, prophylaxis of migraine, allergic disorders.

Adverse reactions: Anticholinergic side effects like dry mouth, blurring of vision, sedation, GI upset and oculogyric spasms.

Contraindications: Urinary retention, glaucoma, hypersensitivity, asthma, neonates, with MAOI.

B. ERGOT ALKALOIDS

Ergotamine

Dose:

- Oral/sublingual dose: 1 mg/dose at onset of attack, may repeat every 30 minutes, till relief (maximum dose: 3 mg)
- IM/SC: 0.25–0.5 mg/dose.

Indications: Migraine, cluster headache, vascular headache, adjuvant in thyrotoxicosis treatment.

Contraindications: Avoid in children <3 years of age, sepsis, ischemic heart disease, peripheral vascular disease, hypertension, liver and kidney disease.

Adverse reactions: Nausea, vomiting, abdominal pain, muscle cramps, weakness, paresthesias, coronary and other vascular spasms.

Dihydroergotamine (DHE)

Adult dose: 2–6 mg oral (maximum 10 mg/day), 0.5–1 mg IM, SC repeat hourly (max 3 mg).

Indication: Migraine

Adverse reactions: Postural hypotension, herpes zoster, mumps.

Dihydroergoloxine (Codegocrine)

Adult dose: 1–1.5 mg oral or sublingual

Indication: Dementia.

Methdilazine Hydrochloride

> 3 years of age dose is 4 mg BD oral.

Indications: Pruritis, neurodermatitis.

Contraindication: Jaundice with levodopa, coma, bone marrow depression.

Pseudoephedrine

Dose:
- <12 years: 4 mg/kg/day q6–8 hr oral
- >12 years: 30–60 mg/dose q6–8 hr

Triprolidine Hydrochloride

Dose:
- 6 months–2 years: 0.3 mg/dose q4–6 hr (maximum: 1.25 mg/day).
- 2–4 years: 0.6 mg/dose q4–6 hr (maximum: 2.5 mg/day)
- 4–6 years: 0.9 mg/dose q4–6 hr (maximum: 3.75 mg/day)
- 6–12 years: 1.25 mg/dose q4–6 hr (maximum: 10 mg/day)

Adult: 2.5 mg/dose q4–6 hr (maximum: 10 mg/day).

Treatment of migraine

Acute migraine:

1. Acetaminophen
   Dose: 15 mg/kg/dose. Side effects: Hepatic necrosis
2. Ibuprofen
   Dose: 7.5–10 mg/kg/dose. Side effects: GI bleeding, stomach upset.

If not relieved, then:

1. Almotriptan (only FDA approved drug in adolescents).
   Dose: 12.5 mg. Side effects: Vascular constriction, serotonin symptoms.
2. Sumatriptan (not approved). Oral: 25, 50, 100 mg
   Nasal: 10 mg and sc 6 mg
   Side effects: Vascular constriction, serotonin symptoms.

PROSTAGLANDINS

PGE1 (Alprostadil)

Dose:

- To keep the ductus arteriosus patent prior to surgery: 0.05–0.4 µg/kg/min.
- After ductus is opened: 0.01 µg/kg/min.

Indication: Ductus dependent congenital heart disease.

Adverse reactions: Platelet aggregation defect, risk of apnea, hypotension.

Contraindication: Persistent fetal circulation.

3

Nonsteroidal
Anti-inflammatory Drugs

NONSELECTIVE COX INHIBITORS

1. Aspirin (Acetylsalicylic acid)

Dose:

- Antipyretic/analgesic: PO/rectal: 10–15 mg/kg/dose q4–6 hr.
- Anti-inflammatory: 60–90 mg/kg/dose oral OR 90–130 mg/ kg/day q4 hr oral.
- Kawasaki disease: 80–100 mg/kg/day q6 hr oral.

Indications: Pain, fever, acute rheumatic fever, Kawasaki disease, prophylaxis against thromboembolism.

Adverse reactions: Hypersensitivity, nausea, vomiting, aspirin toxicity (tinnitus, pruritus, headache).

Contraindications: Bleeding disorders, gout, in children less than 12 years of age or with chickenpox or influenza (Reye's syndrome).

2. Ibuprofen

Dose:

- As antipyretic/analgesic: 5–10 mg/kg/dose q6–8 hr (maximum dose: 40 mg/kg/day).
- Juvenile rheumatoid arthritis: 30–70 mg/kg/day q4–6 hr oral.
- Ductus closure in newborn: 10 mg/kg IV followed by 5 mg/ kg IV every 24 hr for 2 doses.
- Menstrual pain: 200–400 mg q4–6 hr oral.

Indications: Fever, minor aches and pain, juvenile rheumatoid arthritis, cystic fibrosis, ductus closure in newborn.

Contraindications: Salicylate or NSAID allergy, GI bleeding, peptic ulcer disease.

Adverse reactions: Nausea, vomiting, rash, nephrotoxic.

3. Aceclofenac

Avoid in children

Dose: 50–100 mg q12 hrly

Indications: Osteoarthritis, rheumatoid arthritis, ankylosing spondylitis.

Contraindications: Hepatic and renal dysfunction, coronary artery disease, porphyrias, breastfeeding.

Adverse reactions: Dyspepsia, gastric bleeding, gastric ulcer.

4. Diclofenac Sodium

Dose:
- 1–3 mg/kg/day q8 hrly oral
- Avoid IM route in children.

Indications: Rheumatoid arthritis, osteoarthritis, spondylitis, dysmenorrhoea, anti-inflammatory disorders.

Contraindications: Hypersensitivity reactions, gastric bleeding, gastric ulcer.

5. Indomethacin

Dose:
- Rheumatoid arthritis: 1–2 mg/kg/day q8 hrly.
- For ductus closure in premature infants: 0.2 mg/kg/dose q8 hrly IV total 3 doses.

Indications: Closure of patent ductus arteriosus in newborn, rheumatoid disorders, ankylosing spondylitis, gout, Bartter's syndrome.

Adverse reactions: Giupset, frontal headache (most common), leucopenia, rash.

Contraindications: Gastrointestinal lesion or bleeding, asthma, premature infants with necrotizing enterocolitis.

6. Nimesulide

Dose: 5 mg/kg/day q8–12 hrly

Indications: Sinusitis, osteoarthritis, rheumatoid arthritis, ankylosing spondylitis, fever, dental and postoperative pain.

Contraindications: Peptic ulcer, hepatic and renal impairment.

Adverse reactions: Epigastric distress, red colored urine, heart burn, nausea, vomiting, rash.

Avoid in <6 months.

7. Piroxicam

Dose:

- 0.2–0.3 mg/kg/day single dose daily.
- If <15 kg: 5 mg
- 15–25 kg: 10 mg
- 26–45 kg: 20 mg
- >45 kg: 20 mg.

Indications: Juvenile chronic arthritis, rheumatoid arthritis, postoperative pain.

Contraindications: Aspirin/NSAIDs allergy, active peptic ulcer.

Avoid in children <6 years of age.

8. Mefenamic acid

Dose:

Antipyretic: 5–8 mg/kg/dose

Arthritis: 25 mg/kg/day q6–8 hrly orally

Indications: Fever, rheumatoid and osteoarthritis, abdominal pain, dysmenorrhoea.

Contraindications: Gastrointestinal inflammation, peptic ulcer, aspirin allergy.

Adverse reactions: Colitis, seizures, renal damage, GI bleeding.

Avoid in children <6 months.

Do not exceed therapy more than 7 days.

9. Naproxen

Dose:

- Antipyretic: 5–7 mg/kg/dose q8–12 hr

- Juvenile rheumatoid arthritis: 10–20 mg/kg/day q12 hrly orally.

Indications: Juvenile rheumatoid arthritis, fever, pain.

Contraindications: Peptic ulcer disease, GI bleeding, salicylate and NSAID allergy, advanced renal disease.

Adverse reactions: Hepatic and renal toxicity, dyspepsia.

10. Paracetamol

Dose:

- Oral: 15 mg/kg/dose q4–6 hr OR
- 60 mg/kg/day q4–6 hr
- Parenteral: 5 mg/kg/dose IM.
- Rectal: 10–15 mg/kg/dose

Indications: Fever, pain where anti-inflammatory action is not needed.

Contraindications: Hepatic damage, analgesic nephropathy, seizures.

Adverse reaction: Paracetamol toxicity causing hepatic failure, nausea, vomiting.

11. Auranofin

Contains 29% gold.

Dose:

- *Initial dose:* 0.1 mg/kg/day q12 hrly
- *Maintenance:* 0.15 mg/kg/day (maximum dose: 0.2 mg/kg/day).

Indication: Treatment of active stage of rheumatoid and psoriatic arthritis.

Contraindications: Blood dyscrasias, NEC, pulmonary fibrosis, exfoliative dermatitis, bone marrow aplasia.

Adverse reactions: Metallic taste, cloudy urine, dermatitis, stomatitis.

12. Pentazocine hydrochloride

Dose:

- Children >12 years: 50 mg/dose q3–4 hr
- IV/IM dose is 1/3rd of oral dose.

Indication: Moderate to severe pain in surgery, trauma, colic, burns.

Contraindication: Children <12 years, head injury, raised intra-cranial tension, porphyria, respiratory depression.

Adverse reaction: Hepatic toxicity, nausea, sedation.

13. Morphine sulfate

Dose:
- 0.1–0.2 mg/kg/dose sc (maximum dose 15 mg)
- For continuous infusion in neonates: 0.01–0.02 mg/kg/hr and in infants and children: 0.025–0.2 mg/kg/hr

Indications: Preoperative medications, postoperative pain, restlessness, pulmonary edema.

Contraindications: Respiratory depression, coma, seizures, bronchial asthma, head injury, raised intra-cranial tension, acute hepatic disease.

14. Tramadol

It does not produce respiratory depression.
Avoid <14 years of age.

Adult dose: 50–100 mg TDS (maximum: 400 mg/day).

Contraindications: Liver and renal impairment, seizures.

15. Rofecoxib

Adult dose: 25–50 mg/day once or twice a day
Not recommended for children.

Indication: Rheumatoid arthritis.

Dextropropoxyphene hydrochloride

Dose: 2–4 mg/kg/day BD oral

Contraindication: Liver failure.

16. Fentanyl citrate

Dose:
- 0.5–5 µg/kg/dose q1–4 hr iv or as continuous infusion 1–5 µg/kg/hr
- 0.1 mg of fentanyl provides equivalent analgesic effect of 10 mg of morphine.

Sedation: 1–5 µg/kg/dose IV q1–4 hr or as a continuous infusion at 1–5 µg/kg/hr

Oral transmucosal and sublingual: 15–20 µg/kg

Adverse reactions: Skeletal muscle and chest wall rigidity, impaired ventilation, respiratory arrest.

Contraindications: Opioid hypersensitivity, bronchial asthma, respiratory depression, myasthenia gravis, along with MAO inhibitor, <2 years of age.

4

Drugs used for Rheumatoid Arthritis and Gout

A. DISEASE MODIFYING ANTIRHEUMATIC DRUGS (DMARDs)

1. IMMUNOSUPPRESSANTS

a. Methotrexate

Dose:
- Juvenile rheumatoid arthritis: 5–15 mg/m^2/week single dose or 3 divided doses 12 hr apart.
- Antineoplastic dose: 7.5–30 mg/m^2/week oral/IM.

Indication: Juvenile rheumatoid arthritis and other autoimmune diseases.
Choriocarcinoma, acute leukaemias, non-Hodgkin's lymphoma, osteogenic sarcoma.

Contraindications: Bone marrow suppression, renal and hepatic impairment.

Adverse reactions: Megaloblastic anemia, pancytopenia, mucositis, diarrhea, desquamation and bleeding from GIT.

b. Azathioprine

Dose:
- *Kidney transplant:* Initial dose: 2–5 mg/kg/day
  Maintenance dose: 1–3 mg/kg/day oral once a day
- *For rheumatoid arthritis and SLE:* 1 mg/kg/day. Maximum dose 2.5 mg/kg/day for 6–8 weeks.

Indications: Prevention of renal and other graft rejections, rheumatoid arthritis, SLE, steroid resistant nephritic syndrome, inflammatory bowel disease.

Adverse reactions: Bone marrow depression, liver damage, leucopenia, thrombocytopenia, skin cancers, intestinal ulcers, hyperurecemia.

c. Cyclosporin

Dose:

• Prevention of allograft rejection: 10–15 mg/kg/day with milk or fruit juice, gradually reduce to 2–6 mg/kg/day as maintenance for 6 months to 1 year.

• IV dose is 1/3rd of oral dose (5–6 mg/kg) slowly over 2–6 hr

Indications: Prevention of graft rejection in organ transplant, autoimmune diseases, alopecia, corneal transplant, aplastic anemia.

Adverse reactions: Nephrotoxicity, hepatotoxicity, precipitation of diabetes, hyperkalemia, hyperurcemia, opportunistic infections, hirsutism, gum hyperplasia, tremor.

2. SULFASALAZINE

Dose:

• *Ulcerative colitis:* Initial dose: 40–75 mg/kg/day q4–6 hr oral
Maintenance: 30–50 mg/kg/day q4–8 hr oral (maximum 2 g/day).

• *Juvenile rheumatoid arthritis:* 10 mg/kg/day oral

Indication: Juvenile rheumatoid arthritis, ankylosing spondylitis, ulcerative colitis and Crohn's disease.

Adverse reactions: Anaphylaxis, Stevens-Johnson syndrome, leucopenia, agranulocytosis.

Contraindications: Children <2 years, hypersensitivity to sulpha and salicylates, G6PD deficiency, intestinal obstruction.

3. CHLOROQUINE

Chloroquine: 150 and 300 mg (base).

Dose: PO: Acute attack of malaria: Total dose 25 mg base/kg over 3 days, i.e. 10 mg base/kg stat, then 10 mg base/kg at 24 lu and 5 mg base/kg at 48 hr

Prophylaxis: 5 mg base/kg once a week. Start 1 week before exposure and continue for 2–3 weeks after leaving endemic area.

Extraintestinal amoebiasis; PO 10 mg base/kg/day single dose for 2–3 weeks (maximum: 300 mg base/day).

Indications: DOC for prophylaxis of all types of malaria except that caused by resistant *P. falciparum*, extraintestinal amoebiasis, rheumatoid arthritis, discoid lupus erythematous, lepra reactions.

Contraindications: Liver damage, G6PD deficiency, seizure disorder, vision impairment.

Adverse reactions: Hypotension, cardiac depression, arrhythmias, CNS toxicity including convulsions.

Prolonged high dose (as in rheumatiod arthritis, DLE): Loss of vision due to retinal damage.

4. LEFLUNOMIDE

Adult dose: Loading dose of 100 mg daily for 3 days followed by 20 mg OD.

Indication: Rheumatoid arthritis

Contraindication: Children and pregnant/lactating women

Adverse reactions: Diarrhea, headache, rashes, loss of hair, thrombocytopenia, leucopenia, chest infection, raised hepatic transaminases. _

5. GOLD SODIUM THIOMALATE

Dose: Initially 10 mg test dose, then 1 mg/kg/wk for 20 weeks (maximum 50 mg).

Maintenance: 1 mg/kg/dose at 2–4 weeks apart.

Indications: Rheumatoid arthritis, psoriatic arthritis

Contraindications: With antimalarials, immunosuppressive agents, CCf, exfoliative dermatitis

Adverse reactions: Hypotension, stomatitis, kidney and liver damage, bone marrow depression.

6. AURANOFIN

Contains 29% gold

Dose: Initial dose: 0.1 mg/kg/day q12 hrly

Maintenance: 0.15 mg/kg/day (maximum dose: 0.2 mg/kg/day).

Indication: Treatment of active stage of rheumatoid and psoriatic arthritis.

Contraindications: Blood dyscrasias, necrotising enterocolitis, pulmonary fibrosis, exfoliative dermatitis, bone marrow aplasia.

Adverse reactions: Metallic taste, cloudy urine, dermatitis, stomatitis.

7. D-PENICILLAMINE

Dose:
- 20–40 mg/kg/day oral q6–8 hr empty stomach
- Up to 10 years: 0.5–0.75 g/day
- >10 years: 1g/day q12 hr before meals oral
- Give along with vitamin B_6 and zinc.

Adult dose: Start with 125–250 mg OD, then 250 mg BD

Indications: Rheumatoid arthritis, heavy metal poisoning, cystinuria, stage 2 and 3 scleroderma, Wilson's disease

Adverse reactions: Loss of taste, systemic lupus, myasthenia gravis

B. BIOLOGIC RESPONSE MODIFIERS (BRMs)

1. TNF-α INHIBITORS

a. Etanercept

Dose: SC
4–17 years: 0.4 mg/kg/dose (maximum 25 mg) twice weekly, 72–96 hr apart.

Indications: Rheumatoid arthritis, Crohn's disease.

Contraindications: Serious active infection, sepsis.

Adverse reactions: Injection site reaction (pain, redness, itching, swelling), infections like osteomyelitis, pneumonia.

b. Infliximab

Adult dose: 3–5 mg/kg infused IV every 4–8 weeks
Indication: Rheumatoid arthritis.

Adverse reactions: Fever, chills, urticaria, bronchospasm, anaphylaxis, susceptibility to respiratory infections, worsening of CHF.

c. Adalimumab

Adult dose: SC 40 mg every 2 weeks.

Indication: Rheumatoid arthritis

Adverse reactions: Injection site reaction, respiratory infections.

2. IL-1 ANTAGONIST
Anakinra

Adult dose: 100 mg SC daily

Indication: Rheumatoid arthritis

Adverse reactions: Local reactions and chest infections.

C. ADJUVANT DRUGS
Prednisolone

Four times more potent than hydrocortisone.

Dose: 1–2 mg/kg/day q6–8 hr oral after meals.

Indications: All inflammatory disease conditions, allergic conditions, asthma, rheumatic fever, nephrotic syndrome, autoimmune disease, malignancy, pemphigus.

Contraindications: Systemic infection, peptic ulcer, live virus immunization, herpes simplex keratitis.

Adverse reactions: Increased chances of infection, edema, hypertension, hyperglycemia, psychosis, Cushing syndrome, obesity.

DRUGS USED IN GOUT
FOR ACUTE GOUT
1. NSAIDs

(Indomethacin, naproxen, piroxicam, diclofenac or etoricoxib)

Dose: Indomethacin: 3 mg/kg/day q8 hrly

Naproxen: 10–20 mg/kg/day q12 hrly orally

Piroxicam: 20 mg single dose daily

Diclofenac: 1–3 mg/kg/day q8 hrly oral

2. COLCHICINES

Dose:

Acute gout: 0.5–0.6 mg q2 hr till pain is relieved or GI toxicity occurs.

Maximum dose: 8 mg/day.

Indication: Acute and chronic gout.

Adverse reactions: GI toxicity (nausea, vomiting, watery or bloody diarrhoea, abdominal cramps), kidney damage, CNS depression, intestinal bleeding, muscular paralysis and respiratory failure, aplastic anemia, agranulocytosis, myopathy.

3. CORTICOSTEROIDS

Prednisolone:

Four times more potent than hydrocortisone.

Dose: 1–2 mg/kg/day q6–8 hr oral after meals.

Indications: All inflammatory disease conditions, allergic conditions, asthma, rheumatic fever, nephrotic syndrome, autoimmune disease, malignancy, pemphigus.

Contraindications: Systemic infection, peptic ulcer, live virus immunization, herpes simplex keratitis.

Adverse reactions: Increased chances of infection, edema, hypertension, hyperglycemia, psychosis, Cushing syndrome, obesity.

FOR CHRONIC GOUT/HYPERURICEMIA AND URICOSURICS

1. URICOSURIC DRUGS

a. Probenecid

Dose:

- *Loading dose:* 25 mg/kg oral
- *Maintenance:* 40 mg/kg/day q6 hr
- *Maximum single dose:* 500 mg.

Indication: Chronic gout and hyperuricemia

To prolong penicillin or ampicillin action by enhancing and sustaining their blood levels

Adverse reactions: Dyspepsia, rashes, hypersensitivity, convulsion, respiratory failure

Contraindication: Children <2 years, blood dyscriasis, uric acid renal stones.

Advice drink plenty of fluids.

b. Sulfinpyrazone

Adult dose: 100–200 BD

Indication: Chronic gout

Contraindication: Peptic ulcer

Adverse reactions: Gastric irritation, rashes, hypersensitivity reactions.

2. INHIBITOR OF URIC ACID SYNTHESIS
Allopurinol

Dose:
- <10 years: 10 mg/kg/day q8 hr oral
- >10 years: 200–600 mg/day q8 hr oral.

Indication: Chronic gout, secondary hyperuricemia adjunct to chemotherapy of leukemias, Lesch-Nyhan syndrome, Duchenne's muscular dystrophy.

Adverse reaction: Rash, fever, malaise, muscle pain, Stevens-Johnson syndrome, gastric irritation, liver damage, peripheral neuropathy.

Discontinue drug at first sign of rash.

Advice plenty of fluids.

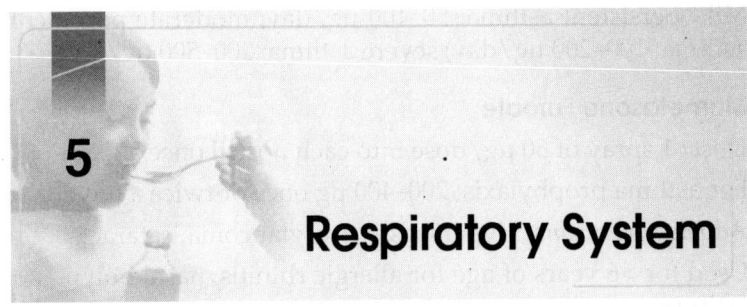

5

Respiratory System

STEROIDS

Beclomethasone Dipropionate

Dose: Inhalation of 200–1000 µg/day in 2 or 4 divided doses.

Mild persistent asthma: 200–400 µg/day; moderate persistent asthma: 400–800 µg/day; severe asthma: 800–1000 µg/day.

Nasal spray: 50 µg metered dose aerosol once or twice a day for allergic rhinitis, vasomotor rhinitis, nasal polyposis.

Adverse reaction: Hoarseness, candidiasis

Budesonide

Inhalation of 100–800 µg/day q12 hr

Mild persistent asthma: 100–400 µg/day; moderate persistent asthma: 400–600 µg/day; severe persistent asthma: 600–800 µg/day.

For croup: 2 mg in 2.5 ml NS BD for 48 hr nebulization.

Ciclesonide

80–160 µg/day.

Not used <12 years of age.

Doxofylline

Above 6 years of age in a dose of 6 mg/kg BD.

Fluticasone Propionate

Usual dose: 50–500 µg/day BD

Mild persistent asthma: 50–100 µg/day; moderate persistent asthma: 100–200 µg/day; severe asthma: 200–500 µg/day.

Mometasone Furoate

Dose: 1 spray of 50 µg/dose into each nostril once a day. For asthma prophylaxis: 200–400 µg once or twice a day.

Adverse reactions: Hypersensitivity, glaucoma, cataracts.

Used for >6 years of age for allergic rhinitis, nasal polyp and asthma.

SYMPATHOMIMETICS

1. Adrenaline

Dose:

• As a bronchodilator: 0.1 ml/kg/dose of 1: 1000 solution im (Maximum dose: 0.5 ml)
• Dose repeated after 15–20 min

Nebulization: 0.25–0.5 ml/kg of 1: 1000 solution diluted in 3 ml of NS.

Indication: Bronchial asthma, anaphylactic shock, cardiac resuscitation.

Adverse reactions: Tachycardia, tremors, hypertension, arrhythmia, angina, tissue necrosis.

Contraindication: Narrow angle glaucoma, brain damage, general anesthesia with cyclopropane.

2. Salbutamol

Dose: PO: 0.1–0.4 mg/kg/dose q8 hrly

Inhalation:

For acute exacerbation: 2–4 puffs of 100 µgs by metered dose inhaler at 20 min intervals followed by 1–2 puffs q4–6 hrly.

Nebulization: 0.15 mg/kg/dose every 20 minutes for 3 doses through a nebulizer using airflow of 6 L/min.

Parenteral: 4–6 µg/kg/dose q6–8 hr sc, im, iv.

Indication: Bronchial asthma, prevention of exercise induced bronchospasm, as an adjunct in treating hyperkalemia in hemodialysis patients.

Adverse reactions: Fine tremors, palpitation, hypokalemia, nervousness, irritability, tachycardia.

Contraindications: Cardiac arrhythmia, shock, hypersensitivity, thyrotoxicosis.

3. Terbutaline

Dose:

Oral: 0.1–0.15 mg/kg/day q8 hrly

SC: 0.005–0.01 mg/kg (maximum: 0.4 mg/dose) q6 hr.

IV: 0.4–1 µg/kg/min (maximum: 10 µg/kg/min)

Inhalation: 1–2 puffs of 250 µg q6–8 hrly

Nebulization:

- <20 kg: 2.5 mg
- >20 kg: 5 mg

Indications: Bronchial asthma, chronic bronchitis, emphysema.

Contraindications: Hypersensitivity to sympathomimetics, arrhythmia, shock.

Adverse reactions: Fine tremors, tachycardia, palpitation, headache, hypokalemia.

4. Bambuterol

Dose: PO

- 2–5 years: 5 mg
- 6–12 years: 10 mg single dose at night.

Used in children above 2 years of age.

Indication: Bronchial (nocturnal) asthma

Contraindicated: Impaired liver function

Adverse reactions: Weakness, nervousness, palpitations, drowsiness.

5. Salmeterol

Dose: Inhalation: 50–100 µg/day (1 puff—25 µg)

Indication: Bronchial asthma (specially in moderate to severe asthma, along with inhaled steroids).

Prophylaxis against allergens and exercise induced asthma, nocturnal asthma.

Contraindications: Children <4 years of age, hypersensitivity reaction, arrhythmia.

Adverse reactions: Nausea, tachycardia, headache, cough.

6. Formoterol Fumarate

Dose: 12 µg inhalation BD

METHYLXANTHINES

1. Theophylline

Dose: 15–25 mg/kg/day q8 hrly oral

Indication: Bronchial asthma (add on therapy in severe asthma)

Contraindications: Hypersensitivity, arrhythmia, peptic ulcer.

Adverse reactions: Toxic level: >20 µg/ml.

GI upset, CNS stimulation: Tremors, nervousness, restlessness, convulsions.

CVS effects: tachycardia, palpitations, hypotension and extra-systoles.

2. Aminophylline

Dose: PO: 15–20 mg/kg/day q8 hrly

Status asthmaticus: Loading dose: 5–7 mg/kg IV

Maintenance: 0.5–0.9 mg/kg/hr IV continuous drip.

Apnea of prematurity: Loading dose: 5 mg/kg iv over 15–20 min.

Maintenance: 2 mg/kg q8 hr oral or IV

Indications: Status asthamaticus, apnea of prematurity, ventilator weaning in neonates, bronchial asthma.

Contraindications: Hypersensitivity, peptic ulcer, seizures.

Adverse reactions: GI upset

CNS stimulation: Irritability, agitation, convulsions, headache

CVS effects: Tachycardia, arrhythmia.

ANTICHOLINERGICS

1. Atropine

Dose:

- For general use: 0.01 mg/kg/dose IV, SC, ET.
- For CPR/sinus bradycardia: 0.01–0.03 mg/kg/dose IV q2–5 min for 2–3 doses.
- For preanesthesia:
  - <5kg: 0.02 mg/kg/dose
  - >5 kg: 0.03 mg/kg/dose

Organophosphorus poisoning: 0.05 mg/kg IV repeat every 5–10 min till atropinization occurs, then repeat dose every 30–60 minutes OR give IV infusion 0.02–0.08 mg/kg/hr.

Inhalation: 0.025–0.05 mg/kg/dose q4–6 hrly (maximum: 2–5 mg/dose).

Indication: Bronchial asthma, reversal of severe bradycardia due to digoxin.

Heart block, antidote for organophosphate poisoning, pre-anesthetic medication, mydriatric and cycloplegic.

Contraindications: Tachycardia secondary to cardiac insufficiency, obstructive gastrointestinal lesions (paralytic ileus, pyloric stenosis), thyrotoxicosis.

Adverse reactions: Arrhythmia, palpitation, delirium, dry, hot skin, tremors, impaired vision.

2. Ipratropium Bromide

Dose:

Nebulization: 250 µg is diluted in 2 ml of normal saline and given over 10 minutes every 20 minutes for 3 doses followed by 250 µg every 2–4 hr

Neonates: 25 µg/kg/dose thrice daily.

Inhalation: 1–2 puffs (1 puff 20 µg) through metered dose inhaler thrice daily.

Indications: Used in combination with B_2 adrenergic agents in bronchial asthma (by inhalation), rhinorrhea, COPD.

Adverse reactions: Tachycardia, drowsiness, blurring of vision, dry mouth, bad taste in mouth.

Contraindication: Hypersensitivity to atropine.

LEUKOTRIENE RECEPTOR ANTAGONIST

1. Montelukast

Dose:

- 2–5 years: 4 mg once a day
- 6–14 years: 5 mg once daily
- >14 years: 10 mg once daily in the evening

Indication: Prophylaxis and treatment of chronic asthma and allergic rhinitis, aspirin sensitive asthmatics.

Contraindication: Acute attack of asthma

Adverse reactions: Palpitations, fatigue, headache, myalgia, raised hepatic enzymes.

2. Zafirlukast

Dose: PO:

- 5–12 years: 10 mg/day q12 hrly
- >12 years: 20 mg/day q12 hrly

Indication: Prophylaxis and treatment of asthma in children >12 years.

Adverse reactions: Headache, upper respiratory infection.

MAST CELL STABILIZERS

1. Sodium Chromoglycate

Dose:

Inhalation: Initial dose: 1–2 puffs (5 mg per MDI) 3–4 times per day OR 1 rotacap (20 mg/cap) 3–4 times/day.

Maintenance: 1 puff 3–4 times/day OR 2–3 rotacaps/day.

Nebulization: 20 mg q6–8 hr

Nasal: 1 spray 3–4 times a day.

Eye: 1–2 drops 3–4 times/day in >4 years

Indications: Prophylaxis of chronic asthma, prevention of allergic rhinitis, vernal keratoconjunctivitis.

Contraindication: Acute asthma

Adverse reactions: Nausea, headache, nasal congestion.

2. Ketotifen

Start at a low dose and increase to maximum of 1 mg BD.

Indications: Prophylaxis of bronchial asthma, symptomatic treatment of allergic rhinitis, conjunctivitis.

ANTITUSSIVE AGENT

1. Codeine

Dose: Antitussive—0.2 mg/kg/dose q8 hrly

For analgesia: 0.5–1 mg/kg/dose q4 hrly oral.

Indications: Dry cough, mild to moderate pain, symptomatic relief of diarrhea.

Contraindications: Liver disease, respiratory depression, bronchial asthma, head injury, raised intracranial pressure.

Adverse reactions: Constipation, sedation, vomiting, anorexia. Advice plenty of fluid and fibre intake to avoid constipation.

2. Dextromethorphan

Dose:
- 1–2 mg/kg/day q8 hr oral (maximum dose: 60 mg/day).
- 2–6 years: 2.5–7.5 mg PO q8 hrly
- 7–12 years: 5–10 mg PO q8 hrly
- >12 years: 10–30 mg PO q8 hrly

Indication: Dry cough, nonketotic hypergylcemia.

Adverse reactions: Vomiting, drowsiness, dizziness.

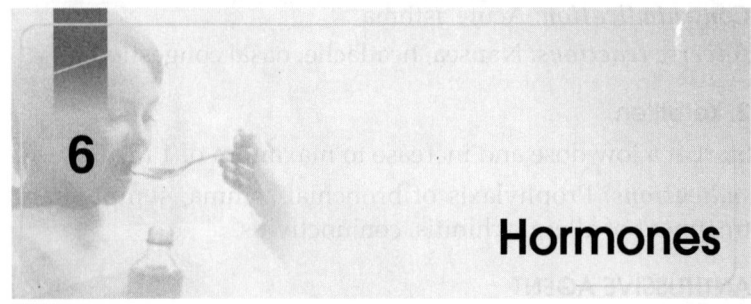

6

Hormones

THYROID HORMONE
L-thyroxine Sodium
Dose: PO single dose on empty stomach.

Newborn babies: 10–15 µg/kg/day
Infants: 6–8 µg/kg/day
1–3 years: 5–6 µg/kg/day
5–10 years: 4–5 µg/kg/day
>10 years: 2–3 µg/kg/day

TSH monitoring: In newborn babies it is done every month till 6 months and then every 2–3 months till 2 years of age.

Indications: Hypothyroidism, cretinism, nontoxic goiter, myxoedema coma, papillary carcinoma of thyroid.

Contraindications: Adrenal and myocardial insufficiency.

Adverse reactions: Tremors, sweating, nervousness, palpitations, tachycardia.

Tri-iodothyronine
25 µg tablet: Not freely available in India

Dose: 0.5–1.5 mg/kg/day single oral dose

For hypothyroid coma: 5–20 mg IV BD.

Indication: Occasionally used IV along with L-thyroxine in myxoedema coma.

THYROID HORMONE SYNTHESIS

A. INHIBIT HORMONE SYNTHESIS (ANTITHYROID DRUGS)

1. Propylthiouracil

Dose: PO
- 1–4 mg/kg/day
- < 10 years: 50–150 mg/day q8 hr
- > 10 years: 150–300 mg/day q8 hr

Maintenance dose: 50 mg BD

Indications: Hyperthyroidism, thyrotoxic crisis.

Contraindication: Agranulocytosis.

Adverse reactions: Vertigo, hepatitis, leucopenia, rash, aplastic anemia.

2. Methimazole

Dose:

Initial dose: 0.25–1 mg/kg/day once a day.

Maximum dose: 30 mg/day.

Maintenance: 1/3rd to ½ of initial dose given along with food.

Indication: Hyperthyroidism.

Adverse reactions: Fever, rash, agranulocytosis, pancytopenia.

3. Carbimazole

Dose:

1–2 mg/kg/day q8 hr oral.

Indications: Thyrotoxicosis prior to surgery, hyperthyroidism.

Contraindications: Tracheal obstruction, nodular goiter, de Quervain's thyroiditis.

Adverse reactions: Urticaria, loss of hair and taste, bone marrow suppression, agranulocytosis.

B. THYROID HORMONE RELEASE

1. Iodine

Dose: Used in adults

Lugols solution: 5% iodine in 10% pot. Iodide solution

Indications: Preoperative preparation for thyroidectomy 5–10 ml TDS oral.

Thyroid storm: 50–100 mg BD oral

Endemic goitre prophylaxis: 20 mg of potassium iodide.

Antiseptic

Adverse reaction: Swelling of lips, eyelids, angioedema of larynx, petechial hemorrhages, thrombocytopenia, lymphadenopathy.

2. Potassium Iodide

Dose:

- 1 ml saturated Lugol's iodine solution/day q8 hr oral OR
- Potassium iodide 50–150 mg/day q8 hr oral.

Indications: Preoperative preparation for thyroidectomy, thyroid storm, endemic goiter prophylaxis, antiseptic.

INSULIN

Dose:

Diabetes mellitus: Insulin range: Toddlers: 0.2–0.4 unit/kg/day

Prepubertal: 0.5–0.8 unit/kg/day

Adolescents: 0.8–1.5 unit/kg/day.

Diabetic ketoacidosis: start with 0.1 unit/kg/hr continuous infusion in normal saline with the help of infusion pump till blood sugar comes down to 300 mg/dl. Switch over to N/2 saline in 5% dextrose and give 0.25 units/kg regular insulin every 1–2 hr before stopping infusion and then every half an hour before meals sc.

Indications: Insulin and noninsulin dependent diabetes mellitus, diabetic ketoacidosis (diabetic coma), hyperkalemia.

Adverse reaction: Hypoglycemia, hypokalemia, lipodystrophy at injection site.

Contraindications: Allergic reactions, insulinoma.

PITUITARY HORMONES

Adrenocorticotropin (ACTH)

Dose:

Immunosuppression/anti-inflammatory: 0.8–1.6 units/kg/day IV/IM q6–8 hr single dose.

Infantile spasms: 20–40 units/day OD IM/SC daily for 4–6 weeks (maximum: 100 units).

Dynamic testing: Short ACTH stimulation test.

<6 months: 62.5 µg; 6 m–2 years: 125 µg; >2 years: 250 µg.

Indications: Infantile spasm, adrenal insufficiency diagnosis, multiple sclerosis exacerbation, muscle weakness in myasthenia gravis.

Adverse reaction: Opportunistic infection, insomnia, nervousness, epistaxis, pancreatitis.

Contraindication: Scleroderma, systemic fungal infection, ocular herpes simplex, peptic ulcer.

Desmopressin

Analoque of vasopressin.

Diabetes insipidus: 5–40 mg once or twice daily intranasal.

Oral: Initially 0.05 mg/dose q12 hr, then gradually increase to 0.08 mg/day.

Nocturnal enuresis: Intranasal 20 µg at bedtime increased to 40 µg. Half dose to be instilled in each nostril.

Oral dose: 0.2 mg at bedtime (maximum: 0.6 mg).

Haemophilia and von Willebrand's type 1.

IV: 0.2–0.4 µg/kg/dose IV diluted in 50 ml NS infused over 15–30 min.

Intranasal: 2–4 µg/kg/dose.

Indications: Treatment of diabetes insipidus, hemophilia, nocturnal enuresis.

Contraindication: Cardiac disease, along with diuretics.

Adverse reactions: Headache, facial flushing, dizziness, hyponatremia, hypertension, water intoxication, seizures.

Somatropin (Synthetic Growth Hormone)

Dose: 0.07–0.1 unit/kg/day SC 6–7 times in a week.

OR 0.18–0.35 mg/kg weekly SC till accepted height is reached.

Turner syndrome/small for gestational age infants: 0.375 mg/kg/week.

Indications: Growth hormone deficiency, neurosecretory dysfunction due to cranial irradiation, chronic renal insufficiency, Turner's syndrome, Prader-Willi syndrome.

Contraindications: Tumor activity evidence, children with closed epiphysis, proliferative retinopathy.

Adverse reactions: Hypothyroidism, lipoatrophy, loss of glycemic control in diabetes, worsening of scoliosis, edema, gynecomastia.

Leuprolide Acetate

Gonadotropin releasing hormone analogue and antineoplastic agent.

Dose:

SC: Start with 35–50 μg/kg/day titrate upward by 10 μg/kg/day.

IM: Start with 0.15–0.3 mg/kg/4 weeks, if downregulation is not achieved then increase by 3.75 mg q4 weeks.

Indication: Central precocious puberty.

Contraindication: Pernicious anemia.

Adverse reaction: Flushing, arrhythmia, bone pain, dysuria, fluid collection at injection site.

Somatostatin

Dose: 1–40 mg/kg/day q2–4 weeks.

Indication: Excess growth hormone.

Adverse reactions: Inhibits gastrointestinal hormonal activity leading to loose stools and nausea.

GLUCAGON

Dose:

- <25 kg: 0.5 mg IM/IV/SC.
- >25 kg: 1 mg IV/IV/SC.

Indications: Treatment of insulin and drug-induced hypoglycemia, hypoglycemia in large for date babies, betablocker poisoining, as a diagnostic aid in radiological examination of GIT.

Contraindications: Small for gestational babies, insulinoma, glucagonoma, pheochromocytoma.

Adverse reactions: Hypersensitivity reactions, tachycardia, hypertension, hypokalemia.

CORTICOSTEROIDS

1. SHORT ACTING
Hydrocortisone

Dose: IV

Anti-inflammatory: 2.5 mg/kg/day q6 hr.

Status asthmaticus: 10 mg/kg/dose stat followed by 5 mg/kg/dose q6 hr.

Shock: 50 mg/kg initial dose followed by 50–150 mg/kg/day q6 hr for 48–72 hrs.

Acute adrenal insufficiency: 50 mg/m^2/day followed by 100 mg/m^2/day. For long-term prophylaxis 10 mg/m^2/day.

Congenital adrenal hyperplasia: 10–15 mg/m^2/day in 3 divided doses.

Indication: Treatment of cortisol insufficiency, status asthmaticus, anaphylactic shock, in newborn for support of blood pressure, meningitis.

Contraindication: Systemic infection, live virus immunization, herpetic or fungal keratitis.

Adverse reactions: Immunosuppression, hypertension, hyperglycemia, Cushing syndrome, cataract.

Abrupt withdrawal causes adrenal insufficiency.

2. INTERMEDIATE ACTING
a. Prednisolone

Four times more potent than hydrocortisone.

Dose: 1–2 mg/kg/day q6–8 hr oral after meals.

Indications: All inflammatory disease conditions, allergic conditions, asthma, rheumatic fever, nephrotic syndrome, autoimmune disease, malignancy, pemphigus.

Contraindications: Systemic infection, peptic ulcer, live virus immunization, herpes simplex keratitis.

Adverse reactions: Increased chances of infection, edema, hypertension, hyperglycemia, psychosis, Cushing syndrome, obesity.

b. Methyl Prednisolone

Dose:

Anti-inflammatory: 0.5–1.7 mg/kg/day IM/IV/oral.

Emergency situations: 30 mg/kg IV bolus over 10–20 minutes, repeat after 4 hours.

Pulse therapy: 30 mg/kg daily for 3–5 days.

Shock: 30 mg/kg/dose q6 hr for 2–3 days.

Status asthmaticus: Loading dose 2 mg/kg/dose IV/IM. Maintenance 2 mg/kg/day q6–8 hr

Indications: Anti-inflammatory and immunosuppressant in idiopathic thrombocytopenic purpura, pulse therapy, asthma, allergic, inflammatory and neoplastic conditions, inflammatory bowel disease.

Adverse reactions: Fluid and electrolyte disturbances, impaired wound healing, fractures, pancreatitis, growth retardation, hypoglycemia.

Contraindications: Systemic fungal infection, live virus immunization.

c. Triamcinolone

Dose: Oral: 24 mg daily QID

Deep IM 40 mg, intra-articular 2.5 = 15 mg.

Indications: Asthma, dermatosis, allergy, adjuvant in leukemia, meningitis, connective tissue diseases, topical anti-inflammatory.

Contraindications: Local/systemic infection, peptic ulcer.

Adverse reactions: Hyperglycemia, myopathy, psychosis, cushing habitus, growth retardation.

Avoid in <6 years age and IV route.

3. LONG ACTING

a. Dexamethasone

Usual dose: 0.05–0.5 mg/kg/day oral.

Anti-inflammatory: 0.08–0.3 mg/kg/day q6 hr

Congenital adrenal hyperplasia: 0.5–1 mg/day oral.

Cerebral edema: 0.5 mg/kg/dose q6 hr IM/IV.

Hib meningitis: 0.6 mg/kg/day q6 hr for 2 days, given prior to or along with first dose of antibiotic.

Pulse therapy: 5 mg/kg iv slow infusion.

For extubation: Newborn; 0.25 mg/kg/dose q12 hr IV for 3–4 doses.

Children: 0.5–2 mg/kg/day q6 hr IV.

Indications: Bronchopulmonary dysplasia, bacterial meningitis, cerebral edema, allergic, autoimmune, inflammatory and neoplastic conditions, enteric fever.

Adverse reactions: Immunosuppression, hypertension, hyperglycemia, hyperacidity, adrenal suppression.

Contraindications: Allergy, diabetes mellitus, psychosis, cardiac failure.

b. Betamethasone

Usual dose:
- 0.1–0.2 mg/kg daily in divided doses oral.
- Up to 1 year: 1 mg; 1–5 years: 2 mg; 6–12 years: 4 mg; adult 0.5–6 mg/day.
- 750 µg is equivalent to 5 mg of prednisolone.
- Fetal lung: 12 mg im 2 doses 24 hrs apart to mother.

Indications: Severe bronchial asthma, fetal lung maturation in <34 weeks gestation, congenital adrenal hyperplasia, cerebral edema, autoimmune disorders.

Adverse reactions: Immunosuppression, delayed wound healing, psychosis, raised ICT, growth retardation, weight gain.

Contraindications: Systemic infection, diabetes, peptic ulcer.

MINERALOCORTICOID

Fludrocortisone

Dose: 0.05–0.2 mg/day oral OD.

Indications: Adrenocortical insufficiency

Adverse reactions: Hypertension, edema, cardiac failure, convulsion, acne, cataract.

Contraindication: Fluid retention, hypokalemia, hypertension, hyperalbuminemia, heart failure.

Deflazacort

Glucocorticoid with anti-inflammatory and immunosuppressive effects.

Dose: 0.25–1.5 mg/kg/day q8–12 hr

Deflazacort 6 mg is equivalent to 5 mg of prednisolone.

ANDROGENS
1. Testosterone (free)

Indication and dose:

Male hypogonadism: 40–50 mg/m^2/dose im every month. *Maintenance:* 100 mg/m^2/dose 2 times/month.

Delayed puberty: 40–50 mg/m^2/dose im every month for 6 months.

Postpubertal cryptorchidism: 10–25 mg 2–3 times/week.

Contraindications: Cardiac, liver, renal impairement.

Adverse reactions: Gynaecomastia, virilization, acne, peliosis hepatitis.

DRUGS AFFECTING CALCIUM BALANCE

CALCIUM
1. Calcium Chloride (27% Ca)

1 g of calcium chloride is equivalent to 273 mg elemental calcium or 13.6 mEq calcium.

Indications and dose:
- Cardiac arrest: 20 mg/kg IV, repeat in 10 min
- Hypocalcemia: 2.5–5 mg/kg/dose IV q4–6 hr
- Hypocalcemic tetany: 10 mg/kg IV over 5–10 min, repeat in 6–8 hr

2. Calcium Gluconate (9% Ca)

1 g of calcium gluconate is equivalent to 89 mg elemental calcium or 4.49 mEq calcium.

10% solution contains 100 mg/ml of calcium gluconate equivalent to elemental calcium of 8.9 mg/ml or 0.45 mEq/ml.

Usual dose: 1–2 ml/kg/dose IV, repeat, if necessary

Maintenance: 2–4 ml/kg/day q6 hr or IV continuous.

Hypocalcemia: 1–2 ml/kg slow IV push.

Cardiac arrest: 0.2–0.5 ml/kg IV.

Hyperkalemia: 0.5 ml/kg over 5–10 min.

Indication: Treatment of symptomatic hypocalcemia, hyperkalemia, cardiac arrest, chronic renal failure.

Adverse reactions: Hypercalcemia, bradycardia, arrhythmia if used with digitalis, tissue necrosis.

Contraindications: Renal calculi, hypophosphatemia, hypercalcemia.

IV solution is diluted to 50 mg/ml and be given slowly over 1 hr under monitoring.

3. Calcium Dibasic Phosphate (23% Ca)

1 g of calcium phosphate is equivalent to 390 mg elemental calcium or 19.3 mEq calcium.

Neonates: 20–80 mg/kg/day q8 hr.

Children: 45–65 mg/kg/day q6–8 hr.

Indication: Calcium deficiency states, rickets, chronic renal failure.

Calcium carbonate used for treatment of hyperphosphatemia.

VITAMIN D

Vitamin D Cholecalciferol

- 1 mg calciferol is equal to 40000 IU, i.e. 10 µg is equal to 400 units.
- For deficiency states: 6,00,000 IU IM single dose or 60,000 IU daily for 10 days or weekly for 10 weeks oral.
- If no healing line is seen on X-ray after 4 weeks, repeat the course.

Maintenance dose: 400 IU per day oral.

Indication: Rickets, osteomalacia, hypoparathyroidism, prophylaxis in conditions leading to vitamin D deficiency.

Adverse reactions: Hydrocephalus, pseudotumor cerebri, nephrocalcinosis.

Contraindications: Hypercalcemia, hypervitaminosis D, decreased renal function.

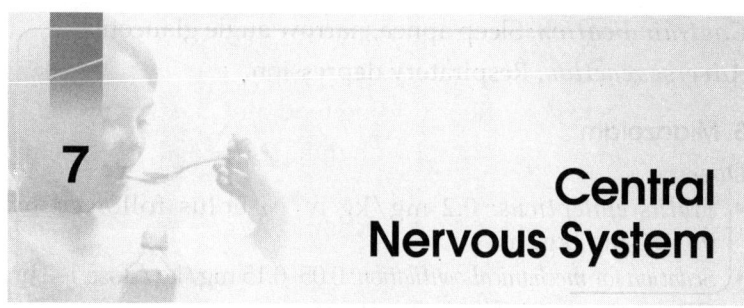

7

Central Nervous System

1. Diazepam

Indication and dose:

In status epilepticus: >1 month: 0.2–0.5 mg/kg/dose IV, may repeat at 3–5 min interval.

- <5 years: 5 mg (maximum dose)
- >5 years: 10 mg (maximum dose)

Per rectal dose: 0.5–0.75 mg/kg/dose.

Neonatal tetanus: 0.5–5 mg/kg IV every 2–4 hr IV (maximum 60 mg/kg/day).

Prophylaxis of febrile seizures (DOC): 0.1 mg/kg/day q8 hr oral, initiate treatment at the first sign of fever and continue for 24 hr after fever is gone.

Anxiety, sedation and muscle relaxation: 0.1–0.3 mg/kg/day q4–8 hr oral.

Contraindication: Myasthenia gravis, acute narrow angle glaucoma, paralytic ileus.

Adverse reaction: Apnea, respiratory depression, hypotension.

2. Lorazepam

Dose: 0.05–0.1 mg/kg by IV/IM, over 2–5 min may repeat once after 10–15 min.

Maximum dose: 4 mg

For sedation: 0.05 mg/kg/dose q4–8 hr oral/IV/IM

Indication: Drug of choice in status epilepticus, used in myoclonus.

Contraindication: Sleep apnea, narrow angle glaucoma.

Adverse reaction: Respiratory depression.

3. Midazolam

Dose:

- *Status epilepticus:* 0.2 mg/kg IV/IM bolus followed by 0.1–0.2 mg/kg/hr
- *Sedation for mechanical ventilation:* 0.05–0.15 mg/kg/dose 1–2 hr
- OR continuous infusion at rate of
  - *For neonates:* 0.2–1 µg/kg/min
  - *For infants and children:* 0.5–3 µg/kg/min
- *Intranasal:* 0.3 mg/kg

Indication: Sedation, status epilepticus.

Contraindications: Respiratory depression, shock, coma, acute narrow angle glaucoma.

Adverse reaction: Hypotension, bradycardia.

4. Valproic Acid

Dose:

- For refractory seizures: 10–15 mg/kg/day 8–12 hr oral (maximum dose: 60 mg/kg/day)
- Therapeutic level: 50–100 mg/L
- In status epilepticus: 20 mg/kg loading dose followed by 5–10 mg/kg/dose 8 hr
- Infuse over 1 hr up to maximum of 20 mg/min.

Indication: GTCS, myoclonic, atypical absence, clonic and tonic seizures.

Bipolar disorders, alternative to carbamazepine intrigeminal neuralgia.

Adverse reaction: Hepatotoxicity in <3 years of age, weight gain, alopecia, tremors

Contraindication: Active liver disease, urea cycle disorders.

5. Paraldehyde

Dose: 0.1–0.2 ml/kg/dose deep IM or 0.3 ml/kg/dose by rectal route mixed with 3:1 coconut oil.

Indication: Uncontrolled status epilepticus.

Adverse reaction: Respiratory depression

Contraindication: Pulmonary and hepatic diseases.

6. Phenytoin

Dose: Status epilepticus:

Loading dose: 15–20 mg/kg slowly IV at 1 mg/kg/min diluted with NS.

Maintenance dose: 5–8 mg/kg/day 8–12 hr or single dose

Anticonvulsant: PO: 15–20 mg/kg 3 times a day.

Maintenance: 5–8 mg/kg/day.

Therapeutic level: 10–20 mg/L.

Indications: GTCS, partial seizures, Class Ib antiarrhythmic drug, status epilepticus, migraine.

Adverse reaction: Hirsutism, gingival hyperplasia, fetal hydantoin syndrome and cerebellar syndrome, megaloblastic anemia.

Contraindication: Porphyria, heart block.

7. Fosphenytoin

Dose:

Loading dose: 15–20 mg/kg IV

Maintenance dose: 4–6 mg/kg/day IV/IM

Maximum IV infusion: 3 mg/kg/min

Indication: Status epilepticus, GTCS, partial seizures.

Contraindication: Porphyria.

Fast infusion can lead to arrhythmia, cardiovascular collapse and coma.

8. Phenobarbitone

Dose:

Loading dose: 15–20 mg/kg IV over 15–20 min at 1 mg/kg/min as slow IV bolus. Additional 5 mg/kg every 15–30 minutes (maximum 30 mg/kg).

Maintenance dose: 3–5 mg/kg/day 12 hrly or single dose at night oral/IV.

Therapeutic level: 15–40 mg/L.

Indication: Neonatal seizures, GTCS, partial seizures, febrile seizure prophylaxis

Contraindication: Porphyria, bradycardia.

Adverse reaction: Sedation, hypotension, respiratory depression.

9. Phenobarbital

Indication and dose:

Status epilepticus: Loading dose: 15–20 mg/kg OD or BD IV.

Anticonvulsant: <1 year: 5–6 mg/kg/day.

- 1–5 years: 6–8 mg/kg/day
- 6–12 years: 4–6 mg/kg/day
- >12 years: 1–3 mg/kg/day IV/oral

Sedation: PO/IM: 2 mg/kg TDS.

Adverse reactions: Tremor, insomnia, liver damage.

Contraindications: Porphyria, CNS depression.

10. Propofol

Indication and dose:

Induction of anesthesia: 1.5–2.5 mg/kg IV.

Maintenance of anesthesia: 9–15 mg/kg/hr IV.

Sedation: 1.5–3 mg/kg/dose over 1–2 min IV.

11. Lignocaine

Indication and dose:

Topical: Maximum dose 3 mg/kg/dose; do not repeat within 2 hr.

Local anesthetic: Maximum dose: 4.5 mg/kg/dose

Arrhythmia: Loading dose: 1 mg/kg/dose IV bolus, continuous infusion: 20–50 µg/kg/min (maximum 5 mg/kg/min).

Postherpetic neuralgia: Apply patch to affected areas, maximum 3 patches.

Contraindication: Cardiac decompensation, AV block, supraventricular arrhythmias.

Adverse reactions: Lethargy, coma, seizures, respiratory depression.

12. Carbamazepine

Dose: 10–30 mg/kg/day; started at 30% to 50% of initial target dose and increased every 5–7 days.

Indications: DOC Partial seizures, trigeminal neuralgia, bipolar disorder, antidiuretic in diabetes insipidus.

Adverse reactions: Headache, ataxia, vertigo, diplopia, aplastic anaemia, hepatotoxicity.

Contraindications: AV conduction defects, bone marrow suppression, porphyria.

13. Ethosuximide

Dose: 15 mg/kg/day q12 hr

Maintenance: 20–40 mg/kg/day q12 hr

Maximum dose:
- <6 years: 500 mg/day
- >6 years: 1500 mg/day

Indication: Absence seizure

Adverse reaction: Photophobia, leukopenia, drowsiness, nausea.

14. ACTH

Dose: 30–40 U/day IM/SC for 4 weeks followed by gradual tapering doses over next 2 weeks.

Indications: Infantile spasm, West syndrome

Contraindications: Cushing syndrome, tuberculosis, fungal infections.

15. Clonazepam

Dose: 0.01–0.03 mg/kg/day q8–12 hr oral. Increase every 3 days by 0.25–0.5 mg till maximum dose of 0.2 mg/kg/day is reached.

Indications: Add on therapy for atonic, akinetic, resistant absence seizures.

Adverse reactions: Fatigue, somnolence, hypotonia, excessive secretions.

Contraindications: Liver disease, narrow angle glaucoma.

16. Lamotrigine

Dose:

- Without valproate: 5–10 mg/kg/day q12 hr oral
- With valproate: 0.5–5 mg/kg/day 24 hr oral.
- With enzyme inducing antiepileptic drug: Start with 2 mg/kg/day and increase to 5–15 mg/kg/day q12 hrly.

Maximum dose: 15 mg/kg/day OR 400 mg/day.

Indications: Add on therapy for absence seizures, myoclonic seizures, depressive phase of manic depressive psychosis, partial seizures, Lennox-Gastaut syndrome. First line drug for absence seizures.

Contraindication: Hepatic disease.

Adverse reactions: Life threatening hypersensitivity skin rash, Stevens-Johnson syndrome and toxic epidermal necrolysis.

17. Topiramate

Dose: Start with 1 mg/kg/day gradually increase to 5–10 mg/kg/day q12 hr or single dose.

Migraine prophylaxis: One half the dose.

Indications: Add on therapy for GTCS, partial seizures, Lennox-Gestaut syndrome.

Adverse reactions: Weight loss, renal stones, somnolence and fatigue.

18. Vigabatrin

Dose: Initial dose: PO: 20–40 mg/kg/day

Maintenance: 80–100 mg/kg/day q8–12 hr

Indications: DOC for infantile spasms. Add on drug for resistant partial seizures, Lennox-Gestaut syndrome.

Adverse reaction: Irreversible visual field defects due to retinal atrophy.

19. Levetiracetam

Dose:
- 4–12 years: Start at 10 mg/kg/day q12 hr; increase by 10 mg/kg/week up to 30 mg/kg/day.
- >12 years: Start at 10 mg/kg/day q12 hr; increase by 10 mg/kg/week up to 1.5 g twice a day.

Indications: Add on drug for partial seizures, absence seizures, myoclonus.

Adverse reactions: Sedation, dizziness, weakness and rarely behavioral changes.

20. Zonisamide

Dose: 4–8 mg/kg/day; 2 doses

Indications: Add on drug for refractory partial seizures, atypical absence seizures.

Adverse reactions: Somnolence, dizziness, headache, renal stones.

21. Clobazam

Dose: 0.1 mg/kg/day
Maintenance dose: 0.3–1 mg/kg/day at bedtime 12 hr.

Prophylaxis of febrile seizures: 1 mg/kg/day q12 hr for 2 days.

Indication: Add on therapy for complex partial seizures, GTCS, absence seizures, febrile seizures prophylaxis.

Contraindication: Myaesthenia gravis.

Adverse reactions: Constipation, weight gain, sleep disturbances.

22. Oxcarbazepine

Dose: Start at 8–10 mg/kg/day BD to a maximum dose of 30 mg/kg/day (up to 1.8 g/day).

Increase by increments of 10 mg/kg/week.

Indication: First line drug for treatment of simple and complex seizures. Add on drug for partial seizures and GTCS.

Contraindication: Use with caution in renal failure.

Adverse reactions: Fatigue, headache, dizziness, ataxia, hyponatremia and skin rash.

23. Acetazolamide

Dose: For refractory seizures and glaucoma, raised intracranial pressure: 8–30 mg/kg/day

Diuretic: 5 mg/kg/day q8 hr

Hydrocephalus: PO: 50–70 mg/kg/day q8 hour

Indication:

• Refractory Seizures and Glaucoma as Diuretic

• Hydrocephalus

• To alkalinize urine in UTI, acute mountain sickness.

Contraindications: Hepatic and renal insufficiency, sodium and potassium depletion.

Adverse reactions: Drowsiness, Hypokalemia, Hyperglycemia, metabolic acidosis, renal calculi.

24. Nitrazepam

Dose: 0.25–1 mg/kg/day q12 hr or single oral dose.

Indications: Myoclonic, absence, partial seizures, infantile spasms, insomnia.

Contraindications: Myasthenia gravis, porphyria and narrow angle glaucoma.

25. Gabapentin

Loading dose: 15 mg/kg/day q8 hr increase over several days to 30–60 mg/kg/day q8 hr.

Indications: Add on therapy for partial and generalized seizures, diabetic neuropathy, postherpetic neuralgia, migraine, neuropathic pain.

Adverse reactions: Somnolence, dizziness, vomiting, tremors.

Avoid below 12 years.

26. Paraldehyde

Dose: 0.1–0.2 ml/kg/dose deep IM or 0.3 ml/kg/dose by rectal route mixed with 3 : 1 coconut oil.

Indication: uncontrolled status epilepticus.

Adverse reaction: Respiratory depression

Contraindication: Pulmonary and hepatic disease.

27. Chlorpromazine

Dose: As antipsychotic, antiemetic; PO, IV, IM: 0.5–1.0 mg/kg/ dose q6–8 hr

Maximum dose:

- 1–5 years: 40 mg/day
- 5–12 years: 75 mg/day.

Chorea: 50 mg/day till chorea is contolled increase by 25 mg/ day. Maximum dose: 300 mg/day.

Neonatal tetanus: 1–2 mg/kg/dose 2–4 hourly.

Amphetamine toxicity: 1 mg/kg IV/IM. Maximum dose: 50 mg.

Indication: Drug of choice for intractable hiccups.

Chorea, agitation, antipsychotic, mania, drug induced and postoperative nausea and vomiting, neonatal tetanus.

Adverse effect: Postural hypotension, tachycardia, weight gain, cholestatic jaundice, extrapyramidal reactions like tardive dyskinesia, dystonia, dry mouth.

Contraindication: Avoid in children <1 year.

Bone marrow depression, coma, severe CNS depression.

28. Haloperidol

Infantile spasm: 0.025–0.05 mg/kg/day.

Psychotic disorder: 0.05–0.15 mg/kg/day.

Behavior disorder: 0.05–0.075 mg/kg/day.

Agitation/chorea: 0.01–0.03 mg/kg/day.

Gilles de la Tourette syndrome: 0.05–0.075 mg/kg/day in 2–3 divided doses.

Adverse reactions: Extrapyramidal and oculogyric reactions (DOC: Benztropine and dimenhydramine); tachycardia, bronchospasm, visual disturbances, anemia.

Contraindications: Severe toxic CNS depression, coma, parkinsonism.

Not recommended for 3–12 years of age.

29. Lithium

Dose: 15–60 mg/kg/day q6–8 hr oral.

Indications: DOC for prophylaxis of bipolar disorder; Prophylaxis of manic-depressive psychosis, treatment of mania, depression, OCD, cancer chemotherapy induced leucopenia.

Contraindications: Renal and cardiac disease, dehydration, hypothyroidism, dyselectrolytemia.

Adverse reactions: Impaired taste, weight gain, tremors, diabetes insipidus.

Maintain blood level: 0.6–1.5 mEq/L

Acute mania: 0.8–1.2 mEq/L

Toxic level: >1.5 mEq/L

Seizures: >2.5 mEq/L

30. Trifluoperazine

Dose: >6 years: 1 mg oral q12–24 hr (maximum: 15 mg/day).

Indications: Hallucination, delusion, agitation, conduct disorder, childhood schizophrenia.

Contraindications: Extrapyramidal reactions, drowsiness, liver and renal disease.

Adverse reactions: Hypotension, arrhythmia, dystonia, constipation.

31. Imipramine

Children: 1.5 mg/kg/day q8 hr oral increase by 1–1.5 mg/kg/day every 3–4 days.

Maximum: 5 mg/kg/day

Adolescents: 25–50 mg/day q6–8 hr oral. Maximum: 100 mg/day

Enuresis: 10–25 mg oral at bedtime gradually increase 10–25 mg/dose at 1–2 weeks interval until desired effect is reached. Continue for 2–3 months, then taper slowly. When dry for 14 consecutive months, give medication on alternate days for 14 days.

Depression: 1.5 mg/kg/day in 2–4 divided doses increase by 1 mg/kg/day every 3–4 days up to 5 mg/kg/day.

Contraindications: Heart block, severe liver disease, along with MAO inhibitors.

32. Amitriptyline

Depression/hyperactivity: 1 mg/kg/day q12 hr, increase to 1.5 mg/kg/day till desired effect is reached.

Nocturnal enuresis: <12 years: 10–25 mg

>12years: 25–50 mg at bedtime for 8 weeks.

Migraine prophylaxis: 0.1–0.25 mg/kg/dose at bedtime slowly increase every 2 weeks by 0.25 mg/kg. Maximum: 2 mg/kg/dose.

Indications: Depression, anxiety, analgesia for neuropathic pain, enuresis.

Adverse reactions: Postural hypotension, arrhythmia, drowsiness, confusion, tremor, weight gain.

Contraindications: Liver and cardiac disease, along with MAO inhibitors.

33. Nortriptyline

Indication and dose:

Depression (6–12 years): 1–3 mg/kg/day q6–8 hr oral.

Nocturnal enuresis: oral 30 minutes before bedtime.

20–25 kg: 10 mg; 25–35 kg: 10–20 mg; 35–54 kg: 25–35 mg

Adverse reactions: Postural hypotension, tachycardia, xerostomia, urinary retention, tremor.

34. Fluoxetine

Dose: >5 years: 5–10 mg oral OD. Maximum dose: 20 mg/day.

Indications: OCD, depression, anxiety, panic disorder, mood stabilizer.

Adverse reactions: Headache, nervousness, anxiety, insomnia, anorexia.

Not recommended below 5 years.

35. Melatonin

Dose: 3 mg 20–30 min before desired sleep time gradually increase dose to 6 mg after 7–10 days for desired response.

Indications: Chronic sleep disturbance in those with neurodevelopmental disabilities like cerebral palsy, autism, visual impairment.

Contraindication: Not recommended below 3 years, epilepsy.

Adverse reactions: Hallucination, hypotension

36. Pemoline

Dose: 1 mg/kg/day oral OD every morning, increase the dose by 0.5 mg/kg/day every 1–2 weeks. Maximum dose: 3 mg/kg/day.

Indications: CNS stimulant in attention deficit hyperactivity disorder, narcolepsy.

Adverse reactions: Loss of weight and appetite, insomnia.

37. Ketamine

Dose:

- IV: 0.5–2 mg/kg at rate not exceed 0.5 mg/kg/min
- IM, oral, rectal: 3–10 mg/kg/dose

Nasal and sublingual: 3–5 mg/kg/dose

Sedation: 2 mg/kg.

Sedation in ventilated patients: Continuous IV infusion at rate of 5–20 µg/kg/min.

Minor procedures: 0.5–1 mg/kg.

Adverse reactions: Hallucinations, purposeless movements of limbs, raised ICT, hypertension, retrograde and antegrade amnesia, increased respiratory secretions, bad dreams.

Contraindications: Raised ICT, cardiac failure.

38. Clonidine hydrochloride

Dose: Neonates for narcotic withdrawal: 1 µg/kg every 6–8 hours maximum: 2 µg/kg/dose q4 hr.

ADHD: 0.05 mg/day increase by 0.05 mg/day every 3–7 days. Maximum: 0.4 mg/day.

Sedation: 4 mg/kg intranasal.

Clonidine tolerance test: 4 µg/kg, single dose—test for growth hormone release from pituitary.

Indications: Sedation, ADHD, hypertension, migraine prophylaxis, Gilles de la Tourette.

Taper dose gradually to avoid symptoms of sympathetic overactivity.

39. Triclofos sodium

Stable ester of trichloroethanol.

Dose: 20 mg/kg/dose oral.

1–5 years: 250–500 mg; 6–12 years: 0.5–1 g

Indications: Sedation, teething, recurrent colic with persistent crying, difficult feeding.

Contraindications: Liver, cardiac and renal impairment.

Adverse reactions: Nausea, headache, skin rash.

40. Thiopental

Loading dose: 5–10 mg/kg IV over 2–5 min

Maintenance dose: 2–10 mg/kg/hr continuous infusion.

Indications: Uncontrolled status epilepticus, mechanical ventilation.

41. Primidone

Dose:
- Newborn: 12–20 mg/kg/day q6–12 hr
- <8 years: 10–25 mg/kg/day q8–12 hr; >8 years: 125–1500 mg/day oral (maximum: 2 g/day).

Therapy is initiated at one-third to half of initial dose.

Indication: Partial and tonic clonic seizures.

42. Lacosamide

Loading dose: 1 mg/kg/day BD

Maintenance dose: 2–12 mg/kg/day BD.

Indications: Adjunct in case of refractory partial onset epilepsy, diabetic neuropathy.

Adverse reactions: Headache, nausea, vomiting, dizziness, ataxia, tremors, diplopia, fatigue, somnolence.

43. Trifluperidol

Dose: 5–12 years: Initial dose is 0.25 mg/day increased slowly over a few days to 2 mg/day.

Acute psychosis: 0.5–2.5 mg IM.

44. Pimozide

Loading dose: 1–2 mg/day in divided doses.

Maintenance dose: 0.2 mg/kg/day or total dose of 10 mg/day.

Maximum dose: 0.3 mg/kg/day or 20 mg/day.

Indications: Paranoid states, Gilles de la Tourette syndrome.

45. Methylphenidate

Initially 5 mg once or twice a day on empty stomach, then gradually increase to a maximum of 60 mg/day.

Severe cases combine with clonidine: 1–4 µg/kg/day OD in the evening.

Indications: Narcolepsy, ADHD, pain.

Contraindication: <6 years of age, glaucoma, along with MAO inhibitors.

Adverse reactions: Anxiety, anorexia, tremors, tachycardia, hypertension, seizures, delayed growth.

·46. Atomoxetin

Dose: 0.5 mg/kg/day increase every week to a maximum of 1.2 mg/kg once or twice a day.

Indication: Nonstimulant medication for ADHD.

Contraindication: <6 years of age.

Adverse reactions: Dizziness, drowsiness, vertigo, anorexia, loss of weight, liver damage.

47. Caffeine Citrate

Indication: Apnea of prematurity.

Loading dose: 10–20 mg/kg slow IV infusion over 30 minutes.

Maintenance dose: 5 mg/kg/day IV over 10 minutes once daily or can be given oral.

Adverse reactions: Necrotizing enterocolitis.

48. Baclofen

Dose:

- 0.75–2 mg/kg/day q8 hr oral.
- Maximum dose: <8 years: 40 mg/day; >8 years: 60 mg/day.

Indication: To relieve muscle spasticity due to spinal or cerebral origin.

MISCELLANEOUS

IMMUNOGLOBULIN

1. Tetanus Immunoglobulin

Dose in newborn: If mother has not received TT, then give 250 IU IM stat.

Children: Prophylaxis: 250 IU IM may increase to 500 IU.

Therapeutic: 500–3000 IU IM.

Indications: Treatment of active cases of tetanus, prophylaxis of those cases in whom immunization status is uncertain like burns, injuries.

Adverse reactions: Soreness at injection site, fever, edema, nephritic syndrome.

2. Tetanus Antitoxin

Prophylactic: 300–5000 units SC, IM.

Therapeutic: 10,000 units IM/IV.

Intrathecal: 250 units q24 hr for 3 injections.

Indication: To provide temporary passive immunity when tetanus immunoglobulin is not available, to neutralize toxin produced by *Clostridium tetani.*

Adverse reactions: Hypersensitivity reactions, hypotension, dyspnea, urticaria, serum sickness.

Test dose should always be given to rule out hypersensitivity.

3. Hepatitis B Immunoglobulin

Newborn: 0.5–1 ml or 100–200 IU IM within 24 hr after birth on anterolateral aspect of thigh.

Children: 0.06 ml/kg or 40 units/kg IM within 24 hr after exposure.

Active immunization with Hepatitis B vaccine to be given simultaneously.

Indication: Prophylaxis in neonates for hepatitis born to HBsAg positive mothers.

Prophylaxis after exposure by accidental needle stick injury, etc.

Adverse reactions: Mild pain, itching at injection site.

4. Human Rabies Specific Immunoglobulin

Recommended for all patients with animal bite who are at risk of developing rabies.

Dose: 20 IU/kg infiltrated locally as much as possible at exposure site. If any remains give it IM at a different site (gluteal or lateral aspect of thigh) within 24 hr presentation.

If patient presents within 1 to 7 days give total dose IM.

Equine immunoglobulin: 40 IU/kg.

Indications: All injuries, licks on mucus membrane by wild animals suspected to be suffering from rabies.

Adverse reactions: Muscle soreness at injection site, tenderness, fever.

Contraindication: Do not administer in repeated doses once vaccine treatment has been initiated.

5. Equine Rabies Specific Immunoglobulin

Equine immunoglobulin: 40 IU/kg
- Intradermal skin testing to be done prior to its administration.
- Infiltrate total dose around the wound, any remaining dose is given IM at gluteal region.
- Used when human rabies immunoglobulin is not available.

Adverse reactions: Serum sickness, hypersensitivity.

6. Human Normal Immunoglobulin

Prophylaxis:
- For 10% solution 0.4 ml/kg IM
- For 16.5% solution 0.25 ml/kg IM

Therapeutic: For 10% solution: 0.6 ml/kg IM

For 16.5% solution: 0.4 ml/kg IM.

Primary immunodeficiency disorders: 300–400 mg/kg IM once q3–4 weeks.

Measles: 0.3 ml/kg IM within 6 days of exposure.

Hepatitis A: 0.02–0.04 ml/kg IM within 14 days of exposure.

Indications: Treatment and prophylaxis of viral diseases, bacterial infections, burns and immunodeficiency disorders.

Contraindication: Selective IgA deficiency hypersensitivity.

Adverse reactions: Flushing with chills, nausea, headache.

7. Human High Dose Immunoglobulin

Dose:

- Ampoules of Intraglobin is available as 5 ml (250 mg), 10 ml (500 mg), 20 ml (1g)
- Infusion bottles as 50 ml (2.5 g), 100 ml (5g), 200 ml (10 g).
- Immunodeficiency and prophylaxis against infections: 2 ml/kg every 3–4 weeks
- Life threatening infections: 3 ml/kg IV daily for 2 days.

Chronic ITP: 8 ml/kg daily for 5 days or 800 mg/kg IV single dose.

Kawasaki disease: 2 g/kg single dose IV infusion over 10–12 hr

Indication: Treatment and prophylaxis of life threatening infections, immunodeficiency states and chronic ITP, Kawasaki disease, GBS, demyelinating polyneuropathy, Rh isoimmunization.

Adverse reactions: Tachycardia, flushing with chills, nausea, dyspnea.

8. Diphtheria Antitoxin

Dose: Pharyngeal and laryngeal diphtheria of 48 hr duration: 20,000–40,000 IU IV.

Nasopharyngeal involvement: 40,000–60,000 IU IV.

Extensive disease of 3 or more days with neck swelling: 80,000–1,20,000 IU IV.

Antitoxin is diluted in 1:20 isotonic sodium chloride solution at 1 ml/min over 60 min.

Diphtheria antitoxin is given to all suspected cases of diphtheria.

Schick test positive contacts: In one arm one dose of diphtheria toxoid and in other arm 500–2000 units of diphtheria antitoxin IM. Give 3 doses of diphtheria toxoid 6 weeks later at monthly interval.

Indications: Passive immunization in suspected cases of diphtheria. And neutralization of toxin produced by *Corynebacterium diphtheriae.*

Adverse reactions: Hypersensitivity reactions and serum sickness.

9. Antisnake Venom

It contains a mixture of four lyophilized polyvalent antisnake serum of common krait, cobra, Russel's viper and saw scaled viper.

It is most effective when given within 1–4 hr, more than 24 hr is used only in severe poisoning.

Dose: Minimum envenomation give 20–50 ml (5 vials)

Moderate cases give 50–150 ml (5–15 vials) and severe cases give 150–200 ml (15–20 vials)

Infusion rate is 20 ml/kg/hr.

Smaller children may require additional 50% (one and half times) dose.

Prophylactically steroids and antihistaminics are used.

Indication: Bites of viperidae and elaipidae.

Adverse reactions: Hypersensitivity reactions, serum sickness, neurological effects.

Contraindication: Hypersensitivity to equine antisera.

10. Varicella Immunoglobulin

Dose: 125 units/kg IM within 48 hr or 96 hr of exposure to varicella OR 0.2–1 ml/kg diluted in NS and administered IV over 1 hr.

Indication: Immunocompromised children, postnatally exposed infants of susceptible mothers.

11. Respiratory Syncytial Virus Immunoglobulin

Dose: 750 mg/kg IV q30 days

Start at 1.5 ml/kg/hr for 15 minutes, increase to 3 ml/kg/hr for 15 minutes. Maximum dose 6 ml/kg/hr.

Indication: RSV infection in <2 years of age with history of prematurity and bronchopulmonary dysplasia, prophylaxis in severe immunodeficiency or immunosuppression.

Colony stimulating factors

Granulocyte colony stimulating factor

Neonates: 5 µg/kg/day for 3–5 days once daily.

Children: 5–10 µg/kg/day once daily for 14 days.

Indication: Cancer patients receiving drugs associated with neutropenia and fever; treatment of congenital or idiopathic neutropenia.

Granulocyte mononuclear colony stimulating factor.

Dose: Neonates: 5–10 µg/kg/day SC once daily for 5 days.

GM-CSF in children: 250 µg/kg as a 2 hr infusion IV or SC once daily for 21 days.

Indication: Neutropenia associated with cytotoxic therapy or after bone marrow transplantation, neutropenia associated with severe HIV disease or sepsis.

Erythropoietin-r Hu

Chronic renal failure: Initially 50–100 IU/kg with maintenance of 10 IU/kg 2–3 times/week IV/SC.

Anemia of prematurity: 150–500 IU/kg twice a week for 8–12 weeks SC.

Give iron supplements 2–3 mg/kg/day.

Indications: Chronic renal failure, neoplasia, anemia of prematurity, chemotherapy induced, associated with AIDS and its therapy.

Adverse reactions: Seizure, headache, hypertension, edema, arthralgia.

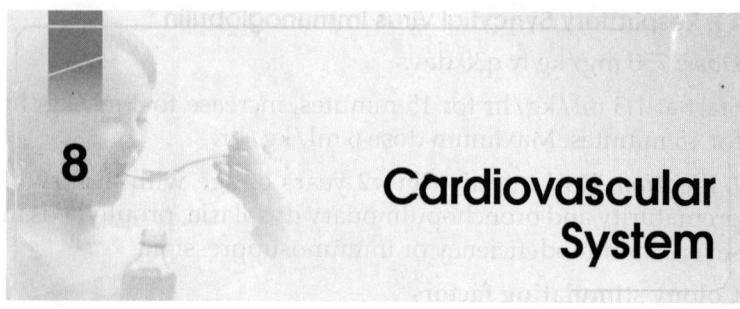

8

Cardiovascular System

INOTROPHIC DRUGS

Digoxin

Dose: PO:

- For premature infants: 20 µg/kg/day
- For full-term neonates: 30 µg/kg/day
- Infants (1 m–12 m): 0.06–0.08 mg/kg/day
  - <2 years: 40–50 µg/kg/day
  - >2 years: 40 µg/kg/day
- Parenteral dose is 2/3rd of this dose.
- One-half of digitalizing dose is given stat followed by 1/4th after 8 hr, and 1/4th after 16 hr.
- Maintenance dose is 1/4th of initial digitalizing dose.

Indications: CCF, atrial fibrillation and flutter, premature beat, paroxysmal supraventricular tachycardias.

Contraindications: Ventricular fibrillation, constrictive pericarditis, HOCM, AV block.

Adverse reactions: Sinus bradycardia, arrhythmia, hypokalemia.

GI symptoms: Anorexia, nausea, vomiting (MC)

Ocular: Blurring of vision, diplopia, photophobia.

Amrinone

Dose: 0.75 mg/kg IV bolus over 2–3 min, then 2–20 µg/kg/min continuous infusion.

0.5 µg/kg IV bolus followed by 2–20 µg/kg/min infusion

Indications: Low cardiac output states, cardiac failure, now withdrawn due to toxicity.

Adverse reactions: Hypotension on iv administration, myocardial infarction, thrombocytopenia.

Dopamine

Dose: 2.5 µg/kg/min iv continuous infusion increased slowly to 20 µg/kg/min.

Maximum dose 50 µg/kg/min.

Indications: DOC for cardiogenic shock or shock not responding to fluid therapy, chronic refractory CCF, low dose in renal failure, dilated cardiomyopathy.

Contraindication: Pheochromocytoma, VF/VT

Adverse reactions: Nausea, vomiting, angina, palpitation, arrhythmia, tissue necrosis.

Dobutamine

Dose: 5–20 µg/kg/min iv continuous infusion. Maximum dose: 40 µg/kg/min.

Indication: Hypotension after adequate fluid therapy, cardiogenic shock, chronic refractory CCF, dilated cardiomyopathy.

Contraindication: Arrhythmia, constrictive pericarditis, HOCM.

Adverse reactions: Tachycardia, palpitation, ectopic beats, tissue necrosis.

ANTIANGINAL

NITRATES

1. Glyceryl trinitrate

Dose:
- Initially 0.25–0.5 µg/kg/min gradually increase by 0.5–1 µg/kg/min every 3–5 min.
- Maximum 20 µg/kg/min.

Indications: CHF, shock, portal hypertension prophylaxis, hypertensive emergencies.

Contraindications: Acute myocardial infarction, closed angle glaucoma, constrictive pericarditis.

Adverse reactions: Headache, halitosis, methemoglobinemia, reflex tachycardia, hypotension, syncope.

2. Isosorbide Dinitrate

Not recommended in children.

Dose: 0.1 mg/kg/day q6–8 hr oral

Maximum dose: 2 mg/kg/day.

Indications: Angina pectoris, intractable congestive cardiac failure.

Contraindications: Acute myocardial infarction, severe asthma

Adverse reactions: Lupus like syndrome, dizziness.

BETA BLOCKER
Propranolol

Indication and dose:

Hypertension/Arrhythmia:

Oral: 0.5–1 mg/kg/day q6–8 hr. (maximum dose: 4 mg/kg/day).

IV: 0.01–0.1 mg/kg/dose over 10–15 min. Maximum dose in infants is 1 mg and 3 mg in children.

Cyanotic spells: 2–6 mg/kg/day q6–8 hr oral

Migraine prophylaxis: 0.6–2 mg/kg/day oral q6–8 hr. Maximum dose: 4 mg/kg/day.

Thyrotoxicosis: 2 mg/kg/day q6–12 hr oral.

Adverse reactions: Lethargy, cold clammy skin, bradycardia, hypotension, hypoglycemia, bronchospasm.

Contraindications: CCF, bronchial asthma, heart block.

CALCIUM CHANNEL BLOCKERS
1. Nifedipine

Dose:

• 0.6–0.9 mg/kg/day oral q6–8 hr
• 10–60 mg orally, sublingually, sr

Indications: Chronic stable angina, hypertension, hypertensive emergencies, HOCM, migraine prophylaxis.

Adverse reactions: Headache, flushing, tachycardia, hypotension.

Contraindication: Cardiogenic shock

2. Diltiazem

Dose: 1.5–2 mg/kg/day oral q6–8 hr

Indications: Hypertension, atrial fibrillation or flutter, supraventricular tachycardia

Adverse reactions: Hypotension, bradycardia, CHF, hepatic injury

Contraindication: 2nd and 3rd degree heart block, sick sinus syndrome

ANTIHYPERTENSIVES

ACE INHIBITORS

1. Captopril

Dose:

Neonates: 0.05–0.1 mg/kg/dose q8–24 hr oral. Maximum dose: 0.5 mg/kg/day.

Children: 0.3–0.5 mg/kg/dose q8–12 hr oral. Maximum dose: 6 mg/kg/day.

Indications: Hypertension, CCF, crisis in scleroderma.

Adverse reactions: Neutropenia, agranulocytosis, cough, angioedema, acute renal failure.

Contraindications: Aortic stenosis, renal impairment.

2. Enalapril

Dose: 0.1–0.6 mg/kg/day q12–24 hr oral.

Indications: Hypertension, CCF.

Adverse reactions: Fatigue, hypotension, cough, hyperkalemia, angioedema.

Contraindications: Aortic stenosis, B/L renal artery stenosis, GFR <30 ml/min/m^2

Rashes, neutropenia, altered taste, cough may be present.

3. Lisinopril

Dose: Children >6 years of age: 0.07 mg/kg/day OD. Maximum: 5 mg.

Indications: Hypertension.

Contraindications: Aortic and renal artery stenosis, hyperkalemia, renal dysfunction.

4. Ramipril

Dose: 2.5–6 mg/m^2 OD.

Indication: Hypertension.

Adverse reactions: Headache, fatigue, dizziness, angioedema.

Contraindication: Hypersensitivity with any ACE inhibitor.

BETA-BLOCKERS

1. Atenolol

Dose: 0.5–2 mg/kg/day OD oral.

Indications: Hypertension, arrhythmias

Contraindication: Bradycardia, heart block, bronchial asthma (rarely), cardiac failure.

2. Propranolol (Non-selective)

Indication and dose:

Hypertension/arrhythmia:

Oral: 0.5–1 mg/kg/day q6–8 hr (maximum dose: 4 mg/kg/day).

IV: 0.01–0.1 mg/kg/dose over 10–15 min. Maximum dose in infants is 1 mg and 3 mg in children

Cyanotic spells: 2–6 mg/kg/day q6–8 hr oral

Migraine prophylaxis: 0.6–2 mg/kg/day oral q6–8 hr Maximum dose: 4 mg/kg/day.

Thyrotoxicosis: 2 mg/kg/day q6–12 hr oral.

Adverse reactions: Lethargy, cold clammy skin, bradycardia, hypotension, hypoglycemia, bronchospasm.

Contraindications: CCF, bronchial asthma, heart block.

3. Labetalol (Alpha + Beta Blocker)

Dose: For hypertensive crisis: 0.25–1 mg/kg IV over 2 minutes, repeat after 5 minutes.

Continuous infusion: 0.4–3 mg/kg/hr

Oral: 5–10 mg/kg/day 12 hrly after meals.

Indication: Hypertensive emergencies.

Adverse reactions: Postural hypertension, rashes

Avoid in asthma, heart failure, hypoglycemia.

4. Carvedilol

• Nonselective beta blocker.

• Dose is not established.

Adult dose: 6.25 mg BD increase to 12.5 mg BD (Maximum: 50 mg/day).

Indications: ADHD, hypertension, prophylaxis of migraine, narcotic withdrawal.

Adverse reactions: Dizziness, dry mouth, drowsiness, fatigue, constipation, rebound hypertension.

CALCIUM CHANNEL BLOCKER

1. Nifedipine

Dose:

• 0.6–0.9 mg/kg/day oral q6–8 hr

• 10–60 mg orally, sublingually, sr

Indications: Chronic stable angina, hypertension, hypertensive emergencies, HOCM, migraine prophylaxis.

Adverse reactions: Headache, flushing, tachycardia, hypotension.

Contraindication: Cardiogenic shock.

2. Verapamil

Dose:

Oral: 2–4 mg/kg/day q8 hr

IV: 0.1–0.4 mg/kg infused over 2 minutes under continuous ECG and BP monitoring.

Indications: Supraventricular tachycardia, extrasystole, hypertension.

Adverse reactions: GI upset, cardiac arrest, hypotension, cardiac arrhythmias.

Contraindications: Cardiogenic shock, AV block, LV dysfunction, sick sinus syndrome.

Avoid in children <2 years of age.

3. Diltiazem

Dose: 1.5–2 mg/kg/day oral q6–8 hr.

Indications: Hypertension, atrial fibrillation or flutter, supraventricular tachycardia.

Adverse reactions: Hypotension, bradycardia, CHF, hepatic injury.

Contraindication: 2nd and 3rd degree heart block, sick sinus syndrome.

4. Amiloride

Dose: 0.4–0.6 mg/kg/day q12–24 hr.

Contraindication: Hyperkalemia, impaired renal function.

Adverse reaction: Nausea, hyperkalemia, anorexia, abdominal pain, flatulence.

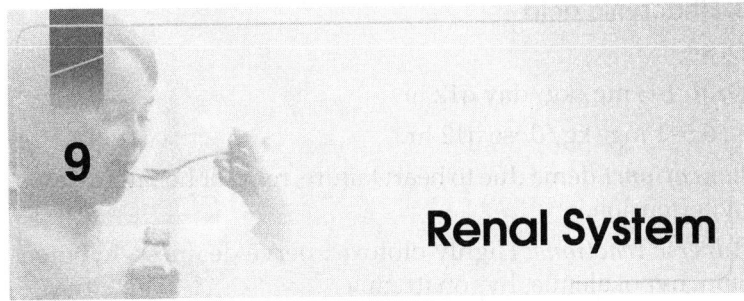

9

Renal System

DIURETICS

LOOP DIURETICS

1. Furosemide

Dose:

Oral: 2–8 mg/kg/day 12 hr. In emergency 1–2 mg/kg/dose q6–8 hr may be given.

IV dose is one-half of oral.

IV infusion rate is 0.1–1 mg/kg/hr

Indications: DOC for moderate to severe renal failure, left ventricular failure, pulmonary and cerebral edema, forced dieresis in poisoning.

Adverse reactions: Hypokalemia, hypomagnesemia, alkalosis, hypotension, thrombocytopenia, hyperuricemia.

Contraindications: Hypovolemia, hypersensitivity to sulphonamides.

2. Bumetanide

Most potent loop diuretic. 40 times more potent than furosemide.

Dose: 0.01–0.02 mg/kg/dose oral.

Indications: Fluid overload secondary to congestive heart failure, hepatic or renal disease.

Adverse reactions: Muscle cramps, gynecomastia, thrombocytopenia, leucopenia.

3. Ethacrynic acid

Dose:

Oral: 1–3 mg/kg/day q12 hr.

IV: 0.5–1 mg/kg/dose q12 hr.

Indication: Edema due to heart failure, renal or hepatic disease, hypertension.

Adverse reactions: Highly ototoxic, nerve deafness, hypotension, hypokalemia, hyponatremia.

THIAZIDES

1. Hydrochlorothiazide

Dose: Oral: 1–2 mg/kg/day q12 hr

Indication: Mild to moderate edema, hypertension, diabetes insipidus, to prevent recurrent renal stones.

Contraindications: Hepatic and renal failure, hypercalcaemia.

Adverse reactions: Hepatitis, leucopenia, hypokalemia, hyponatremia, hyperglycemia.

2. Chlorthalidone

Dose: 1–2 mg/kg/day single dose oral

Indications: Edema, hypertension

Contraindication: Anuria.

3. Metolazone

Dose: Oral: 0.2–0.4 mg/kg/day single daily dose.

Contraindications: Anuria, coma, renal damage.

Adverse reactions: Hypokalemia, hyponatremia, hypotension

CARBONIC ANHYDRASE INHIBITORS

Acetazolamide

Dose: For refractory seizures and glaucoma, raised intracranial pressure: 8–30 mg/kg/day

Diuretic: 5 mg/kg/day q8 hr

Hydrocephalus: PO: 50–70 mg/kg/day q8 hr

Indications:
- Refractory seizures and glaucoma as diuretic
- Hydrocephalus
- To alkalinize urine in UTI, acute mountain sickness.

Contraindication: Hepatic and renal insufficiency, sodium and potassium depletion.

Adverse effect: Drowsiness, hypokalemia, hyperglycemia, metabolic acidosis, renal calculi.

POTASSIUM SPARING DIURETICS

1. Spironolactone

Dose:

Diuretic: Oral-2–3 mg/kg/day OD. Along with thiazides.

Antihypertensive: 1–3.3 mg/kg/day q6–12 hr

Primary hyperaldosteronism: 100–400 mg/m^2/day q12–24 hr

Indications: Hypertension, to counteract potassium loss due to thiazide and loop diuretics.

Adverse reactions: Hyperkalemia, gynecomastia, lethargy, drowsiness, confusion.

Contraindications: Hyperkalemia, anuria, renal failure, Addison's disease.

2. Triamterene

Dose: Oral: 2–4 mg/kg/day q12 hr

Indications: Edema associated with cardiac failure, cirrhosis, nephritic syndrome, as an adjunct to other diuretics, hypertension.

Contraindications: Hyperkalemia, renal failure, liver disease.

Adverse reactions: Headache, constipation, hyponatremia, acidosis.

OSMOTIC DIURETICS

Mannitol

Dose:
- Raised intracranial pressure/brain edema: Initially 5 ml/kg thereafter 2 ml/kg every 6 hr for 2 days IV rapidly over a period of 30–60 minutes.

• For oliguria: 10% of dose over 3–5 minutes and rest during next 2–6 hr.

Indications: To reduce intracranial pressure, to maintain GFR and urine flow in acute renal failure.

Contraindications: Acute tubular necrosis, anuria, cerebral hemorrhage, pulmonary edema.

Adverse reactions: Headache, electrolyte imbalance.

10 Hematological System

COAGULANTS
A. Vitamin K
a. *K1 Fat soluble*
   i. Phytonadione

Dose:
- Hemorrhagic disease of newborn prophylaxis: 1 mg for term and 0.5 mg for preterm IM.
- Therapeutic dose: 2.5–5 mg/dose IV/IM/SC. Maximum dose: 10 mg.

Indications:
Dietary deficiency, prolonged antimicrobial therapy, bleeding tendency due to liver disease, hemorrhagic disease of newborns prophylaxis, prevention and treatment of hypoprothrombinemia due to deficiency of vitamin K dependent clotting factors, antidote of dicoumarol and warfarin poisoining.

Contraindication: Coagulation disorders.

Adverse reactions: Breathlessness, chest constriction, fall in BP

b. *K3 (Synthetic)*
   i. *Fat soluble*
   - Menadione
   - Acetomenaphthone
   ii. *Water soluble*
   - Menadione sodium bisulphate
   - Menadione sodium diphosphate

B. Desmopressin

Indication and dose:

Hemophilia and von Willebrand's disease: 0.2–0.4 µg/kg/dose IV diluted in 50 ml NS given over 15–30 minutes.

Intranasal: 2–4 µg/kg/dose.

Diabetes insipidus:

Oral: Start with 0.05 mg/dose BD, then increase to 0.8 mg/day.

Intranasal: 5–30 µg/day OD/BD.

SC/IV: 2–5 µg/day OD/BD.

Nocturnal enuresis >6 years:

Intranasal: 20 µg/day increased to 40 µg at bedtime. PO: 0.05–0.1 mg at bedtime.

Contraindication: Cardiac insufficiency

Adverse reactions: Facial flushing, headache, tachycardia, hyponatremia.

C. Ethamsylate

Dose:

• Newborn: 12.5 mg/kg IM q6 hr.
• Children: 125–250 mg tds oral/IV

Indications:

• Prevention and treatment of capillary bleeding associated with hematemesis, malena, hematuria, hemoptysis, epistaxis.
• Prevention and treatment of periventricular hemorrhage in newborn.

Contraindications: Porphyria, hemophilia.

Adverse reactions: Nausea, rash, headache, transient hypotension.

ANTICOAGULANTS

A. Parenteral Drugs

i. Heparin

Indication and dose:

For thrombosis: Loading dose: 50 units/kg IV

Maintenance dose: 10–25 units/kg/hr as continuous IV infusion OR 50–100 units/kg/dose q4 hr IV

May give double dose as loading dose and maintain prothrombin time between 1.5 and 2.5 times of control.

DVT prophylaxis: 5000 units/dose SC q8–12 hr until ambulatory.

For catheter patency: 1–2 ml of heparin solution (10 units/ml) every 4–6 hr

For total parenteral nutrition and arterial line flushing: 0.5–1 units/ml.

Other indications: Prophylaxis and treatment of pulmonary embolism, peripheral arterial embolism, DIC, TIA.

Contraindication: Bleeding disorder, thrombocytopenia.

Adverse reactions: Bleeding from various sites, hypersensitivity reactions.

ii. Low Molecular Weight Heparin (LMWH): Enoxaparin

Dose: SC

<2 months prophylaxis: 0.75 mg/kg/dose q12 hr. Treatment: 1–5 mg/kg/d q12 hr.

>2 months–<18 months prophylaxis: 0.5 mg/kg/dose q12 hr. Treatment: 1 mg/kg/dose q12 hr

Indications: DIC, purpura fulminans, prophylaxis and treatment of thromboembolism.

Contraindications: Bleeding disorder, GI ulcer.

Overdose is treated with protamine sulfate.

B. Oral Drugs

a. Coumarin Derivatives

i. Warfarin sodium

Loading dose: 0.2 mg/kg OD followed by 0.1 mg/kg/day OD.

Maintenance range: 0.05–0.34 mg/kg/day oral/parenteral.

Target prothrombin time: 2–3 INR.

Indications: Treatment and prophylaxis of venous thromboembolic disorders, pulmonary embolism; arterial thromboembolism in patient with prosthetic heart valves or atrial fibrillation.

Adverse reactions:
- Hemoptysis, bleeding, skin necrosis.
- Overdose treated with vitamin K

ii. Acenocoumarol

Adult dose: 1–8 mg/day single dose oral. Maintain prothrombin time 1.5 times the normal.

b. Indandione Derivative

Pheninindione

Dose: 0.5–4 mg/kg/day q12 oral.

Indication: Thromboembolism

Contraindication: Bleeding disorder, severe HTN.

ANTI-FIBRINOLYTIC DRUGS

i. Epsilon-amino caproic acid (EACA)

Dose: PO, IV.

Loading dose: 100–200 mg/kg

Maintenance dose: 100 mg/kg q6 hr (maximum 30 g).

In traumatic hyphema: 100 mg/kg q4 hr.

Indications: Treatment of excessive bleeding from systemic hyperfibrinolysis, traumatic ocular hyphema.

Contraindication: DIC

Adverse reactions: Hypotension, seizure, headache, bradycardia, nasal congestion.

ii. Tranexamic acid

Dose:
- IV: 10–15 mg/kg 2–3 times a day
- PO: 25 mg/kg/dose 3–4 times a day.

Indications: Overdose of fibrinolytics, after cardio-pulmonary bypass surgery, prevention of excessive bleeding after tonsillectomy, recurrent epistaxis, ocular trauma, bleeding peptic ulcer.

Contraindication: Intravascular thrombosis.

Adverse reactions: Nausea, diarrhea, headache, giddiness, thrombophlebitis.

ANTI-PLATELET DRUGS

i. Aspirin

Dose:

Antipyretic/analgesic: PO/rectal: 10–15 mg/kg/dose q4–6 hr.

Anti-inflammatory: 60–90 mg/kg/dose oral OR 90–130 mg/ kg/day q4 hr oral.

Kawasaki disease: 80–100 mg/kg/day q6 hr oral.

Indications: Pain, fever, acute rheumatic fever, Kawasaki disease, prophylaxis against thromboembolism.

Adverse reactions: Hypersensitivity, nausea, vomiting, aspirin toxicity (tinnitus, pruritus, headache).

Contraindications: Bleeding disorders, gout, in children less than 12 years of age or with chickenpox or influenza (Reye's syndrome).

ii. Dipyridomole

Dose: 3–6 mg/kg/day in 3 divided doses.

Indication: Prevention of thromboembolic disorders.

Adverse reactions: Dizziness, hypotension.

HYPOLIPIDEMIC DRUGS

A. HGM-CoA Reductase Inhibitors (Statins)

i. Lovastatin

Dose: 10–40 mg/day with evening meal.

Indications:
- Hyperlipoproteinemia
- Primary hyperlipidemia, increased LDL

Contraindications: Diabetes, liver disease

Adverse reactions: Headache, diarrhea, cataract

ii. Pravastatin

Dose:
- 14–18 years: 40 mg/day
- 8–13 years: 20 mg/day.

Indications: Adolescents with heterozygous familial hyper-cholesterolemia.

Contraindications: Active liver disease.

Adverse reaction: Malignancy, cataracts.

iii. Atorvastatin

Dose: 10 mg/day up to maximum of 20 mg for children above 10 years.

B. Inhibit Liposis

Nicotinic acid

Dose: Initially 100–250 mg/day (Maximum 10 mg/kg/day) in 3 divided doses with meals.

Indication: Hyperlipidemia

Contraindication: Peptic ulcer.

Adverse reactions: Flushing, GI upset, pruritus.

PLASMA EXPANDERS

A. Human Albumin

Dose:

Hypoproteinemia: 0.5–1 g/kg/dose IV. Repeat every 1–2 days. Rate of administration should not exceed 2 ml/min over 2–4 hr

Hypovolemia: 0.5–1 g/kg/dose. Maximum 6 g/kg/day. Rapid infusion.

Cerebral edema: 50–80 ml/kg rapid infusion.

Indications: Burns, hypovolemia, hypoproteinemia, plasma volume expansion and maintenance of cardiac output, prior to exchange transfusion in neonatal jaundice, cerebral edema, nephritic syndrome.

Contraindication: Congestive heart failure, severe anemia, pulmonary edema.

Adverse reactions: Fluid overload, congestive heart failure.

Albumin 5% used for hypovolemia and 25% for patients with fluid or sodium restriction.

B. Dextran

    i. Dextran 40

    ii. Dextran 70

Dose is calculated according to patient's condition.

Total dose on day 1 is 20 ml/kg, thereafter 10 ml/kg/day. Do not use for more than 5 days.

Dextran 40:

Indications: Prevention of DVT, shock, cerebrovascular accident.

Contraindication: Fluid overload, renal failure.

Adverse reactions: Anaphylaxis.

Dextran 70:

Indication: For short-term volume expansion and prevention of DVT.

Contraindication: Congestive cardiac failure, bleeding disorder, thrombocytopenia.

Adverse reactions: Anaphylaxis.

C. Degraded Gelatin Polymer (Polygeline)

Haemaccel

Dose: 10–20 ml/kg bolus as rapidly as possible.

Indications: Hypovolemic shock, burns.

11

Gastrointestinal System

PEPTIC ULCER

1. REDUCTION OF GASTRIC ACID SECRETION

a. H$_2$ Antihistamines

i. Cimetidine

Dose:
- 20–40 mg/kg/day every 4–6 hr oral/IV.
- Use in children is limited.

Indication: Duodenal ulcers, stress ulcers, Zollinger-Ellison syndrome, reflux esophagitis.

Adverse reactions: Headache, dizziness, dry mouth, rash, gynecomastia, increase in plasma transaminases.

ii. Ranitidine

Dose: 2–4 mg/kg/day every 12 hr for 4–6 wk oral. IV dose is one-half of oral.

Indication: Duodenal ulcers, gastric ulcers, stress ulcers, gastritis, Zollinger-Ellison syndrome, GERD, prophylaxis of aspiration pneumonia.

Contraindication: Cautious use in renal and liver diseases.

Adverse reactions: Headache, dizziness, bowel upset, rash, confusion.

iii. Famotidine

Dose: 0.4 mg/kg/day at bedtime or 12 hrly.

Indications: Duodenal and gastric ulcers, Zollinger-Ellison syndrome, GERD.

Contraindication: Gastric malignancy.

Adverse reactions: Headache, dizziness, bowel upset, rash, constipation.

b. Proton Pump Blockers

Indications: Duodenal and gastric ulcers, Zollinger-Ellison syndrome, GERD, adjuvant therapy in treatment of *H. pylori* infection, erosive gastritis.

Adverse reactions: Headache, abdominal pain, dizziness, rash, leucopenia.

Pantoprazole: Drug of choice for NSAID induced gastric/peptic ulcer.

Dose: >6 years: 0.5 mg/kg once a day oral.

Omeprazole: *Dose:* >2 years: 0.6–0.7 mg/kg once a day oral.

Lansoprazole: Dose: >1 year: 0.5 mg/kg once a day oral.

Esomeprazole: Dose:
- 1–11 years: 10 mg once daily.
- 12–17 years: 20–40 mg once daily oral.

c. Anticholinergics:

i. Propantheline

Dose: Adults: 15 mg every 8 hr one hr before meals, 30 mg at night. Maximum dose: 120 mg/day.

Children: 1–2 mg/kg/day oral in 3–4 divided doses.

Indications: Peptic ulcer, irritable bowel syndrome, ureteral and urinary bladder spasm, adjunctive therapy of pancreatitis.

Contraindications: Urinary atony, glaucoma, hiatus hernia, reflux esophagitis.

Adverse reaction: Dry mouth, blurring of vision, urinary hesitancy and retention, loss of taste sensation, dizziness.

ii. Oxyphenonium

Dose: 0.8 mg/kg/day q6 hr oral.

Preschool children: 5–10 drops.

Older children: 10–20 drops.

Indication: Antispasmodic

Contraindication: Glaucoma

Adverse reactions: Dry mouth, blurring of vision, urinary retention, dizziness, tremors.

2. NEUTRALIZATION OF GASTRIC ACID
a. Systemic
i. Sodium Bicarbonate

Dose: 7.5% solution is equivalent to 0.9 mEq/ml.

Older children: 1–2 mEq/kg of 7.5% solution.

Subsequent dose is calculated as

Base deficit × weight in kg × 0.6 = mEq or ml of 7.5% solution of sodium bicarbonate.

For IV use dilute in equal volume of sterile water.

Indications: Correction of documented metabolic acidosis during prolonged resuscitation, bicarbonate deficit due to renal or GI losses, to correct acidosis in diabetic ketoacidosis.

Contraindications: Inadequate ventilation, hypernatremia, hypocalcemia.

Adverse reactions: Metabolic alkalosis, hypernatremia, hypocalcemia, local tissue necrosis, pulmonary edema.

ii. Sodium citrate

Dose: 5–15 ml after meals and bedtime or 2–3 mEq/kg/day in 3–4 divided doses.

Indication: Treatment of metabolic acidosis.

Contraindication: Dehydration, anuria, renal impairment, untreated Addison's disease, peptic ulcer.

Adverse reactions: Diarrhea, metabolic alkalosis, bowel obstruction.

b. Nonsystemic
i. Magnesium hydroxide

Dose: PO

Antacid: 2.5–5 ml/dose or 311 mg tablet 4 times a day.

Laxative:
- <2 years: 0.5 ml/kg/dose
- 2–5 years: 5–15 ml/day
- 6–11 years: 15–30 ml/day
- >12 years: 30–60 ml/day.

Indication: Used as a laxative and antacid.

Contraindication: Renal impairment, appendicitis, intestinal obstruction.

Adverse reactions: Chalky taste, diarrhea, prolonged PR interval.

ii. Aluminium hydroxide gel

Dose: PO

Peptic ulcer: 5–15 ml q3–6 hr after meals and at bedtime.

GI bleeding: 5–15 ml q1–2 hr

Hyperphosphatemia
- 50–150 mg/kg q4–6 hr
- 1 gm neutralizes 10 mEq HCl

Indications: Prevention of GI bleeding, peptic ulcer, hyperphosphatemia.

Contraindication: Children <6 years, intestinal obstruction, renal failure.

Adverse reaction: Chalky taste, constipation, urinary calculi.

iii. Calcium Carbonate

Dose: PO: 45–65 mg/kg/day in 3–4 divided doses.

Indication: Hypocalcemia, hyperphosphatemia.

Contraindication: Renal calculi, hypercalcemia, ventricular fibrillation, hypercalciuria.

Adverse reactions: Hypotension, milk-alkali syndrome (headache, decreased appetite, nausea, vomiting, tiredness).

3. ULCER PROTECTIVES

i. Sucralfate

Dose: 40–80 mg/kg/day q6 hr.

Stomatitis: 5–10 ml of 1 g/10 ml, swish and spit or swish and swallow 4 times a day.

Indications: Peptic ulcers, stress ulcers, NSAID associated mucosal damage, topically for chemotherapy induced stomatitis, burns.

Contraindications: Along with antacids, renal dysfunction.

Adverse reactions: Constipation (MC), dry mouth, hypophosphatemia, headache, vertigo.

ii. Colloidal Bismuth Subcitrate (CBS)

Dose: 7–8 mg/kg/day q6 hr oral.

Indication: Chronic gastric and duodenal ulcer resistant to H_2 antagonist.

As an adjunct to treatment of traveller's diarrhea.

Contraindication: Renal failure.

Adverse reactions: Blackening of tongue, black stools, bismuth toxicity (osteodystrophy and encephalopathy), headache.

ANTIEMETIC DRUGS

1. Anticholinergics

i. Hyosine

Dose: 6–12 years: 10 mg q8 hr oral OR 10–20 mg IV/IM bolus.

Indications: Motion sickness prophylaxis, intestinal and biliary colic, adjunctive therapy of peptic ulcer, infant colic, hypermotility of lower urinary tract.

Contraindication: Acute congestive glaucoma, megacolon, GI mechanical obstruction, tachycardia, urinary retention.

Adverse reactions: Dryness of mouth, difficulty in passing urine, blurring of vision.

ii. Dicyclomine

Dose: PO 15 minutes before feed QID (1 ml = 10 mg of dicyclomine).

- <6 months: 5–10 drops
- 6 m–2 years: 10–20 drops
- >2 years: 1 ml

OR >6 months: 5 mg/dose and children: 10 mg/dose.

Indication: Motion sickness prophylaxis, infantile and renal colic, GI and biliary spasms, functional disturbances of GI motility.

Adverse reactions: Headache, dizziness, seizure.

Contraindications: Intestinal obstruction, urinary tract obstruction, glaucoma, tachycardia.

2. H_2 Antihistamines

i. Promethazine

Dose:

- Motion sickness: 0.5 mg/kg/dose q12 hr 30 minutes before start of journey.
- Antiemetic, sedation: 0.25–1 mg/kg/dose q4–6 hr oral/IV/IM/PR.
- Antihistaminic: 0.1 mg/kg/day q6–8 hr and 0.5 mg/kg/dose at night oral.

Indications: Motion sickness prophylaxis, postoperative nausea and vomiting, allergic reactions, sedation.

Adverse reactions: Drowsiness, paraesthesia, tinnitus, blurring of vision.

Contraindication: <2 years, asthma and sleep apnea.

ii. Diphenhydramine

Dose: Extrapyramidal reactions: 1–2 mg/kg IV every 30 min, may be repeated after 3–4 hr IM/oral (maximum dose: 300 mg/day).

- Dry cough: oral q4 hr.
- 2–6 years: 6.25 mg
- 6–12 years: 12.5 mg
- >12 years: 25 mg
- Nighttime sleep: 2–12 years: 1 mg/kg/dose and >12 years 50 mg.

Indications: Motion sickness prophylaxis, antitussive, phenothiazine induced dystonic reactions, nighttime sedation, allergic reactions.

Adverse reactions: Sedation, drowsiness, anticholinergic side effects.

Contraindications: Porphyria.

iii. Dimenhydrinate

Dose: 5 mg/kg/day q6 hr oral/IM/IV.

Maximum dose: 2–6 years: 75 mg/day and 6–12 years: 150 mg/day.

Indications: Vertigo-associated with motion sickness, radiation and chemotherapy-induced nausea, vomiting.

Adverse reactions: Sedation, dizziness, blurring of vision, urinary retention.

Contraindications: Children <2 years.

3. Neuroleptics

i. Chlorpromazine

Dose: 0.5 mg/kg/dose q4–6 hr oral/IM.

Maximum dose:

- 1–5 years: 40 mg/day
- >5 years: 75 mg/day.

Indications: Drug, postoperative, radiation, chemotherapy-induced nausea and vomiting, mania, behavioral problems, neonatal tetanus, to relieve restlessness and apprehension prior to surgery, intractable hiccups.

Caution: Pheochromocytoma, bone marrow suppression, coma.

Adverse reactions: Hypotension, tachycardia, extrapyramidal reactions.

ii. Prochlorperazine

Dose: >2 years/>10 kg: 0.4 mg/kg/day every 8 hr oral. IM dose is half of oral.

Indications: Vertigo-associated vomiting, chemotherapy-induced vomiting.

Contraindications: Liver damage, bone marrow depression.

Adverse reactions: Extrapyramidal reactions, postural hypotension.

4. Prokinetic Drugs

i. Metoclopramide

Dose: GERD/GI dysmotility/galactogogue: 0.1 mg/kg/dose 6–8 hr oral/IM/IV (maximum: 0.8 mg/kg/day).

Chemotherapy induced vomiting: 2–3 mg/kg/dose before and after chemotherapy.

Indications: Nausea and vomiting due to various cases, GERD, gastroparesis, persistent hiccups.

Adverse reactions: Extrapyramidal reactions, hyperprolactinemia leading to galactorrhea, loose motions, tremors.

Contraindications: GI obstruction, pheochromocytoma, epilepsy.

Extrapyramidal reactions are treated with diphenhydramine.

ii. Domperidone

Dose: 0.2–0.4 mg/kg/dose every 4–8 hr oral.

Indication: Nausea and vomiting due to any cause, L-dopa induced vomiting, reflux esophagitis.

Contraindications: GI obstruction and bleeding, liver damage, epilepsy.

Adverse reactions: Arrhythmia, hyperprolactinemia causing gynecomastia in males and galactorrhea in females.

iii. Cisapride

Banned in India from March 2011.

Dose: 0.5 mg/kg/day oral q6–8 hr.

Indication: Previously used for GERD and chronic constipation.

Adverse reactions: Torsades de pointes, ventricular fibrillation.

5. 5HT$_3$ Antagonist

i. Ondansetron

Dose:

- Oral q4 hrs.
- <4 years: 2 mg, 4–11 years: 4 mg and >12 years: 8 mg.
- IV: >3 years 0.15–0.45 mg/kg/dose at 30 min before and 4 and 8 hr after emetogenic drugs.

Indications: Drug of choice for chemotherapy and radiation therapy induced vomiting, prophylaxis and treatment of postoperative nausea and vomiting.

Contraindications: Children <3 years of age, liver damage, prolonged QT interval.

Adverse reactions: Headache, hypotension, bradycardia, allergic reactions.

ii. Granisetron

10–15 times more potent than ondansetron

Dose: >2 years and adult: 10–20 μg/kg/dose IV over 15–60 minutes before chemotherapy, may be repeated 2–3 times after chemotherapy.

OR 40 μg/kg/dose 15–60 minutes before chemotherapy single dose.

Indications: Chemotherapy, radiation and postoperative-induced nausea and vomiting.

iii. Palonosetron

Indication and dose:

• Prophylaxis of postoperative nausea and vomiting: 75 μg single dose immediately before induction of anesthesia.
• Chemotherapy-induced nausea and vomiting: 250 μg single dose.

Contraindication: Intestinal obstruction, ileus.

6. Adjuvant Antiemetics

i. Dexamethasone

Usual dose: 0.05–0.5 mg/kg/day oral.

Anti-inflammatory: 0.08–0.3 mg/kg/day q6 hr.

Congenital adrenal hyperplasia: 0.5–1 mg/day oral.

Cerebral edema: 0.5 mg/kg/dose q6 hr IM/IV.

Hib meningitis: 0.6 mg/kg/day q6 hr for 2 days, given prior to or along with first dose of antibiotic.

Pulse therapy: 5 mg/kg IV slow infusion.

For extubation: Newborn; 0.25 mg/kg/dose q12 hr IV for 3–4 doses.

Children: 0.5–2 mg/kg/day q6 hr IV.

Indications: Bronchopulmonary dysplasia, bacterial meningitis, cerebral edema, allergic, autoimmune, inflammatory and neoplastic conditions, enteric fever.

Adverse reactions: Immunosuppression, hypertension, hyperglycemia, hyperacidity, adrenal suppression.

Contraindications: Allergy, diabetes mellitus, psychosis, cardiac failure.

CONSTIPATION

1. BULK FORMING:
Methylcellulose

Dose:
- 6–12 years: half tbsp (8 g) in 250 ml of cold water OD.
- >12 years: 1 tbsp in 250 ml of cold water 1–3 times daily.

Indication: Laxative.

Contraindications: Abdominal pain, partial bowel obstruction.

Adverse reactions: Abdominal discomfort, cramps, esophageal/bowel obstruction.

2. STOOL SOFTENER
Docusates (DOSS)

Dose:
- <3 years: 10–40 mg/day; 3–6 years: 20–60 mg/day; 6–12 years: 40–150 mg/day
- >12 years: 50–500 mg/day in 1–4 doses oral.

Indications: Constipation, bowel preparation before radiological procedure, to avoid straining during defecation.

Contraindication: Intestinal obstruction.

Adverse reactions: Diarrhea, abdominal cramps.

3. STIMULANT PURGATIVES
a. Diphenylmethanes
i. Bisacodyl
Dose: Oral 0.3 mg/kg/day OD at bedtime or before breakfast. (maximum: 30 mg/day).

Rectal suppository: <2 years: 5 mg; 2–11years: 5–10 mg; >11 years: 10 mg.

Indications: Constipation, X-ray and pre-operative preparation.

Contraindications: Intestinal obstruction, undiagnosed abdominal symptoms.

Adverse reactions: Mucosal irritation, rectal inflammation, abdominal cramps, skin rash.

b. Anthraquinones
i. Senna

Dose: 1–2 tablets hs oral.

Indications: Constipation, bowel evacuation for diagnostic and therapeutic purpose.

Contraindications: Intestinal obstruction, electrolyte imbalance.

Adverse reactions: Diarrhea, nausea, rash.

ii. Cascara sargrada

Dose: Infants: 1.25 ml/day: 2–11 years: 2.5 ml/day; >12 years: 5 ml/day oral at bedtime.

Indication: Constipation

Contraindications: Abdominal pain, intestinal obstruction, CHF.

Adverse reactions: Abnormal discoloration of urine, chronic use would lead to loss of normal bowel function.

Chronic use of senna and cascara may lead to melanosis coli (brown pigmentation of colon).

4. OSMOTIC PURGATIVES
Magnesium Salts
i. Magnesium sulfate
- 50% solution contains 50 mg/ml and provides 4 mEq/ml of elemental magnesium.
- 1% solution contains 10 mg/ml and provides 0.08 mEq/ml of elemental magnesium.

Dose:
- PEM: 2–3 mEq/kg/day
- 0.5–1 ml/kg/day q6 hr IM.

Hypomagnesemia: 25–50 mg/kg/dose q8 hr in neonates and q6 hr in children for 3–4 doses.

Bronchodilator: 25 mg/kg/dose single dose.

Seizures and hypertension: 20–100 mg/kg/dose IV/IM q4–6 hr.

Indications: Osmotic purgative for preparation of bowel before surgery and colonoscopy, any type of poisoning, tapeworm infestation, protein energy malnutrition, convulsions, hypomagnesemia, bronchial asthma, hypertension.

Adverse reactions: Hypotension, hypermagnesemia, abdominal cramps, muscle weakness, CNS depression.

Contraindications: Renal insufficiency.

ii. Magnesium hydroxide

Dose: PO

Antacid: 2.5–5 ml/dose or 311 mg tablet 4 times a day.

Laxative: <2 years: 0.5 ml/kg/dose
- 2–5 years: 5–15 ml/day
- 6–11 years: 15–30 ml/day
- >12 years: 30–60 ml/day.

Indication: Used as a laxative and antacid.

Contraindication: Renal impairment, appendicitis, intestinal obstruction.

Adverse reactions: Chalky taste, diarrhea, prolonged PR interval.

iii. Lactulose

Dose: 1–2 ml/kg/day every 6 hours

Indication: Relief of constipation and fecal impaction, hepatic encephalopathy.

Contraindications: Galactosemia, intestinal obstruction.

Adverse reactions: Diarrhea, abdominal cramps, hypernatremia, bloating.

Advice to drink plenty of fluids.

DIARRHEA

a. Antisecretory Drugs

i. Sulfasalazine

Dose: Initially 40–75 mg/kg/day oral q4–6 hrly.

Maintenance dose: 30–50 mg/kg/day oral q6–8 hrly.

Indication: First line drug for treatment of mild to moderate ulcerative colitis, also used in rheumatoid arthritis.

Contraindication: Hypersensitivity to sulpha and salicylates, children <2 years, G6PD deficiency.

Adverse reactions: Tinnitus, headache, epigastric discomfort, yellowish discoloration of urine and skin, fever with rash.

ii. Mesalazine (Mesalamine)

Different formulations like time release tablets and coating in pH sensitive resins that dissolve at pH 7 are known as mesalamines.

Dose: 50 mg/kg/day q6–12 hrly oral.

Indications: To prevent relapse in ulcerative colitis, also used in proctosigmoiditis and proctitis.

Contraindications: Hypersensitivity to salicylates, renal and hepatic impairment.

Adverse reactions: Abdominal pain/cramps, headache, diarrhea, fever, itching, leucopenia.

iii. Prednisolone

Four times more potent than hydrocortisone.

Dose: 1–2 mg/kg/day q6–8 hr oral after meals.

Indications: All inflammatory disease conditions, allergic conditions, asthma, rheumatic fever, nephrotic syndrome, autoimmune disease, malignancy, pemphigus.

Contraindications: Systemic infection, peptic ulcer, live virus immunization, herpes simplex keratitis.

Adverse reactions: Increased chances of infection, edema, hypertension, hyperglycemia, psychosis, Cushing syndrome.

iv. Racecadotril

It is an enkephalinase inhibitor, thereby preventing loss of water and electrolytes from the intestine.

Dose:

- 1.5 mg/kg/dose 3 times a day.
- Approximate dosage: 2 months–1 year: Half–1 sachet of 10 mg TDS.
- 1–2.5 years: 1.5–2 sachets of 10 mg TDS.
- 2.5–9 years: 1 sachet of 30 mg TDS.
- >9 years: 2 sachets of 30 mg TDS.

Indications: Acute watery diarrhea, diarrhea of bacterial or viral origin, chronic HIV-associated diarrhea.

Adverse reactions: Nausea, vomiting, dizziness, migraine, constipation.

b. Antimotility Drugs

i. Codeine

Dose: Anti-tussive—0.2 mg/kg/dose q8 hrly

For analgesia—0.5–1 mg/kg/dose q4 hrly oral (maximum 60 mg/dose).

Indications: Dry cough, mild to moderate pain, symptomatic relief of diarrhea.

Contraindications: Liver disease, respiratory depression, bronchial asthma, head injury, raised intracranial pressure.

Adverse reactions:

- Constipation, sedation, vomiting, anorexia.
  Advice plenty of fluid and fibre intake to avoid constipation.

ii. Diphenoxylate (Lomotil)

Antiperistaltic agent which inhibits excessive GI motility. Atropine is added to prevent abuse liability.

Dose: PO:

- 2–5 years: 2 mg 3 times a day.
- 6–8 years: 2 mg 4 times a day
- 9–12 years: 2 mg 5 times a day.

Indication: Symptomatic relief of diarrhea.

Adverse reactions: Paralytic ileus, toxic megacolon, anorexia, dizziness, nausea.

Contraindication: Children <2 years of age, dehydration, jaundice, liver disease, pseudomembranous colitis.

iii. Loperamide

Dose: PO

- 2–5 years: 1 mg/dose TDS.
- 6–8 years: 2 mg/dose BD.
- 8–12 years: 2 mg/dose TDS.

Indications: Symptomatic relief of acute and chronic diarrhea, to reduce fluid loss from stomach in patients with colostomies and ileostomies.

Contraindications: Children <2 years of age, constipation, ulcerative colitis.

Adverse reactions: Abdominal distension, toxic megacolon, constipation.

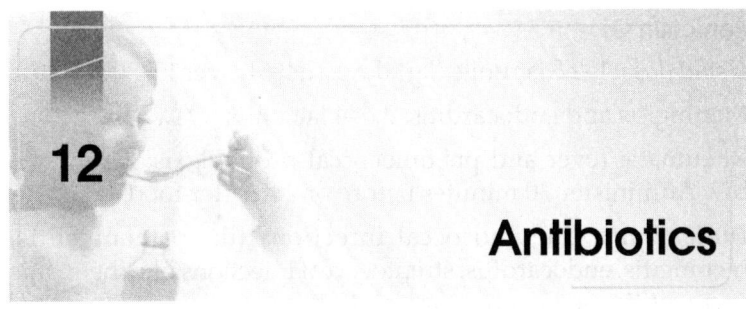

12

Antibiotics

A. AGAINST GRAM-POSITIVE ORGANISMS

PENICILLIN

Carbenicillin

Dose: 400–600 mg/kg/day q4–6 hr IV/IM. IV injection given over 15–30 minutes.

Indications: Infections due to Proteus and Pseudomonas, septicemia, urinary and respiratory tract infections, endocarditis, meningitis.

Adverse reactions: Hypokalemia, hypersensitivity, alteration in platelet function, skin rash.

Caution: Do not use along with digoxin and gentamicin as it causes hypokalemia.

Cloxacillin

Dose:

Staphylococcal infection: 50–100 mg/kg/day q6h oral/IV.

Meningitis: 200 mg/kg/day q4h IV (maximum dose: 4 g/day).

Indications: Active against penicillinase producing staphylococci, mastitis, skin infections, osteomyelitis, pneumonia, endocarditis.

Contraindication: Neonates with jaundice.

Adverse reactions: Hypersensitivity, nausea, thrombophlebitis.

Penicillin G

Usual dose: 1–2.5 lac units/kg/day IM q4–6 h over 15–30 minutes.

Meningitis and endocarditis: 2.5–4 lac units IV/IM q4h.

Rheumatic fever and pneumococcal prophylaxis: 2 lac units BD. Administer 30 minutes before or 2 hr after food.

Indications: Pneumococcal infections like osteomyelitis, meningitis, endocarditis, streptococcal infections like rheumatic fever, otitis media, pneumonia, diphtheria.

Contraindication: Hypersensitivity to penicillin

Adverse reactions: Skin rash, anaphylaxis, neutropenia, Jarisch-Herxheimer reaction, electrolyte imbalance, thrombophlebitis. Advice use penicillin after intradermal testing.

Penicillin G Benzathine

Dose:

- Newborn: 50,000 units/kg IM single dose.
- Prophylaxis of rheumatic fever: <6 years: 0.6 megaunits IM every 3 weeks.
- >6 years: 1.2 megaunits IM every 3 weeks.

Indications: Prophylaxis of rheumatic fever, pneumococcal and glomerulonephritis, diphtheria carriers, streptococcal infections, tetanus.

Adverse reactions: Anaphylaxis, acute interstitial nephritis, convulsions, rash.

CEPHALOSPORINS
Cefazolin

Dose: 50–100 mg/kg/day IV/IM q8 hr.

Newborn:

- <7 days: 40 mg/kg/day BD IV/IM.
- >7 days: 40–60 mg/kg/day q8 hr IV/IM.

Indications: Endocarditis, liver abscess, surgical prophylaxis, genitourinary, respiratory, skin, bone and biliary tract infections.

Contraindications: Pseudomembranous colitis, premature newborn, porphyria.

Adverse reactions: Skin rash, perineal itching, confusion.

Cefuroxime

Oral: 20–30 mg/kg/day BD

IV/IM: 100–150 mg/kg/day q6–8 hr.

Enteric fever: 40 mg/kg/day q12 hr oral.

Indications: Treatment of meningitis caused by meningococci, pneumococci and *H. influenzae*, respiratory tract infections, surgical prophylaxis.

Adverse reactions: Rash, thrombophlebitis, fever, increase in hepatic enzymes.

Cefotaxime

Dose:

Newborn: IV/IM

- <7 days; 100 mg/kg/day q12 hrly
- >7 days; 1200 g: 100 mg/kg/day q12 hrly
- >1200 g; 150 mg/kg/day q8 hrly
- 1 month to 12 yr: IV/IM
- <50 kg: 100–200 mg/kg/day q6–8 hr

Meningitis: 200 mg/kg/day q6 hr

Indications: Broad spectrum active against Gram-positive and Gram-negative bacteria and anaerobes, septicemia, soft tissue infections, intra-abdominal infections, urinary tract infections, osteomyelitis.

Contraindications: Cephalosporin hypersensitivity, renal dysfunction.

Adverse reactions: Pain after IM injection, diarrhea, hypersensitivity reaction, nephrotoxicity.

Cefaclor

Dose: 20–40 mg/kg/day q8 hr oral (maximum dose: 2 g/day).

Indications: Respiratory tract, skin, soft tissue and ENT infections, cystitis.

Adverse reactions: Oral candidiasis, diarrhea, colitis, nephrotoxicity.

Cefadroxil

Dose: 30 mg/kg/day oral BD

Indications: Staphylococcal/streptococcal skin infections, group A beta hemolytic streptococcal pharyngitis, otitis media, urinary tract infection.

Cefdinir

Dose: 14 mg/kg/day oral single or 2 divided doses (maximum dose: 600 mg/day).

Indications: Community acquired pneumonia, chronic bronchitis, maxillary sinusitis, pharyngitis.

Adverse reactions: Nausea, diarrhea, dyspepsia, hypotension, blood dyscrasias.

Cefditoren pivoxil

Dose: 3 mg/kg/dose q8 hr for 5 days for eradication of group *Astaphylococcal hemolyticus.*

Cefixime

Usual dose: 8 mg/kg/day oral once or twice a day.

Enteric fever: 10–15 mg/kg/day once or twice a day oral.

Indications: Pharyngitis, tonsillitis, otitis media, bronchitis.

Adverse reactions: Nausea, diarrhea, genital pruritus, thrombocytopenia, eosinophilia, leucopenia.

Cefoperazone

Dose: 100 mg/kg/day q12 hr IV/IM.

Indications: Septicemia, respiratory tract, urinary tract, skin and soft tissue infections, peritonitis.

Adverse reactions: Rash, urticaria, transient increase in liver enzymes, neutropenia.

Ceftazidime

Dose: 100–150 mg/kg/day IV/IM q8 hr.

Meningitis: 150 mg/kg/day q8 hr IV/IM.

Indications: Active against *Pseudomonas aeruginosa*.

Adverse reactions: Skin rash, thrombophlebitis, pseudomembranous colitis, neutropenia.

Cefpirome

Dose: 30–60 mg/kg/day q12 hr IV.

Broad spectrum including pseudomonas, MRSA, coagulase negative staphylococcal and *Enterococcus faecalis*.

Indications: Severe pneumonia, septicemia, cystic fibrosis, urinary tract infection.

Adverse reactions: Nausea, diarrhea, pseudomembranous colitis, blood dyscrasias, angioedema.

Cefpodoxime

Dose: 10 mg/kg/day BD oral (maximum dose: 400 mg/day). Given along with food.

Indications: Tonsillitis, pharyngitis, bronchitis, pneumonia.

Adverse reactions: Nausea, pruritus, rash, pulmonary eosinophilia.

Cefprozil

Dose: 15–30 mg/kg/day q12 hr

Avoid <6 months of age.

Indications: Pharyngitis, tonsillitis, sinusitis, otitis media, skin infections.

Adverse reactions: Oral candidiasis, diarrhea, coitis.

Cefepime

Dose: <2 months: 60 mg/kg/day; >2 months: 100 mg/kg/day q12 hr IV.

Meningitis, neutropenia: 150 mg/kg/day IV q8 hr.

Indications: Pneumonia, empirical therapy for febrile neutropenia, septicemia.

Adverse reactions: Rash, fever, hypotension, thrombophlebitis, palpitation.

Ceftibuten

Dose: 9 mg/kg/day oral OD.

Indications: Gram-positive and Gram-negative organisms except pseudomonas, enterococcus, enterobacter, chronic bronchitis, otitis media, tonsillitis, pharyngitis.

Ceftizoxime

Dose: 100–200 mg/kg/day IM/IV q6–8 hr

Indications: Lower respiratory tract infection, cellulitis, pyoderma, septicemia.

Adverse reactions: Nausea, rash, candidiasis, phlebitis.

Cephalexin

Dose: 25–100 mg/kg/day oral q6–8 hr

Indications: Sinusitis, otitis media, respiratory, genitourinary, skin, soft tissue and dental infections.

Contraindication: Hypersensitivity to penicillin and cephalosporin.

Adverse reactions: Hypersensitivity, rash, neutropenia, nausea.

Doxycycline (Broad Spectrum Antibiotic)

Dose: 2–5 mg/kg/day BD oral.

Rickettsia: 2.2 mg/kg/dose q12 hr

Indications: Chronic bronchitis, brucellosis, Chlamydia, mycoplasma, rickettsia, cholera, acne.

Contraindication: Children <8 years of age.

Adverse reactions: Nausea, vomiting, diarrhea, phototoxicity, teeth staining.

Vancomycin (Glycopeptide Antibiotic)

Usual dose: 40 mg/kg/day q6 hr IV infusion over 60 minutes.

CNS infections: 60 mg/kg/day q6 hr.

Pseudomembranous colitis: 40–50 mg/kg/day q6–8 hr oral.

Indications: Penicillinase resistant staphylococcal (MRSA) and pneumococcal infections, antibiotic-associated diarrhea.

Contraindication: In renal insufficiency

Adverse reactions: Nerve deafness, skin allergy, hypotension, nephrotoxicity

Red man syndrome: Flushing of face and neck following rapid IV infusion. Give slow IV infusion over 1 hr or administer antihistamines just before infusion.

QUINOLONES
Sparfloxacin
Dose: 4 mg/kg single oral dose.

Indication: Pneumonia, sinusitis, urinary, lower respiratory tract and skin infections, otitis media.

Adverse reactions: Nausea, photosensitivity, tremors.

Limited study on use in children.

Levofloxacin
Dose: 10 mg/kg single dose oral/IV (maximum dose: 500 mg).

Indications: Pneumonia, otitis media, urinary tract infections, MDR tuberculosis.

Contraindication: Along with antacids.

Norfloxacin
Dose: 10–15 mg/kg/day q12h oral.

Indications: Urogenital infections, enteric fever, bacterial gastroenteritis, topical for eye and ear infections.

Adverse reactions: Nausea, heartburn, headache, rash, eosinophilia, neutropenia, thrombocytopenia, tinnitus.

Pefloxacin
Dose: 12 mg/kg/day oral q12h

Indications: Meningitis, septicemia, Gram-negative and Gram-positive organisms, respiratory, urinary, and intra-abdominal infections.

Contraindications: G6PD deficiency, hepatic disease.

Adverse reactions: Nausea, arthralgia, thrombocytopenia, photosensitivity.

Lincomycin

Dose: Oral: 30–60 mg/kg/day q8h

IV/IM: 10–20 mg/kg/day q8–12 hr

Indications: Upper respiratory tract infections, osteomyelitis, topical for acne vulgaris.

Adverse reactions: Pseudomembranous colitis.

Amoxicillin with Clavulanic Acid

- Dose based on amoxicillin component.
- Oral: Newborn: 30 mg/kg/day q12h
- Children: 25–50 mg/kg/day q8–12h
- IV: Newborn: 50 mg/kg/day q12h
- Children: 50–100 mg/kg/day q6–8h

Indications: Broad spectrum antibiotic including beta-lactamase producing strains, tonsillitis, bronchitis, pneumonia, pyelonephritis, lower respiratory, genitourinary, skin and soft tissue infections.

Adverse reactions: Diarrhea, rash, urticaria, pseudomembranous colitis, Candida superinfections.

Contraindications: Penicillin allergy, jaundice, hepatic dysfunction.

Penicillin V (Phenoxymethyl Penicillin)

Dose: 25–50 mg/kg/day q4–8h oral (maximum dose: 3g/day).

- Infants: 62.5–125 mg/dose; <5 years: 125 mg/dose; 6–12 years: 250 mg/dose q6h, given 30 minutes before or 2 hr after meals

For rheumatic fever prophylaxis—<5 years: 125 mg/dose BD oral

- >5 years: 250 mg/dose BD oral.

Indications: Mild to moderate infections caused by Gram-positive and Gram-negative organisms, Lyme disease, pneumococcal prophylaxis following spleenectomy, rheumatic prophylaxis.

Adverse reactions: Vomiting, urticaria, angioedema, neutropenia, thrombocytopenia.

Piperacillin

Dose: 200–300 mg/kg/day q4–6h IV/IM.
- <7 days: 150 mg/kg/day q8–12h IV
- >7 days: 200 mg/kg/day q6–8h IV.

Indications: Infections caused by pseudomonas, *E. coli* bacteroids; neonatal, lower respiratory, intra-abdominal, urinary and bone infections, septicemia.

Adverse reactions: Bleeding, superinfections, thrombophlebitis, headache.

Piperacillin with Tazobactum

- Dose based on piperacillin component.
- 300–400 mg/kg/day IV/IM q6–8h.
- IV infusion is given over 20–30 minutes or IV injection over 3–5 minutes.

Indications: Lower respiratory tract, skin, soft tissue and intra-abdominal infections, appendicitis, peritonitis, organisms that are susceptible to beta-lactamase producing strains.

Adverse reactions: Bleeding, superinfections, diarrhea, headache, colitis.

Contraindications: Hypersensitivity to penicillin, piperacillin, beta-lactum inhibitors.

Procaine Penicillin G

Dose:
- Newborn >1.2 kg: 50,000 units/kg/day IM
- Children: 25,000–50,000 units/kg/day for 10 days IM (maximum dose: 4.8 million units/dose).

Indications: Gonorrhea, syphilis, anthrax, pneumonia, Whipple's disease.

Adverse reactions: Attack of anxiety, agitation, pseudoallergic reactions occur on IV injection.

Avoid IV route.

Ticarcillin with Clavulanic Acid

Dose: 200–300 mg/kg/day IV q4–6h. Maximum: 24 g/day.

Indications: Septicemia, skin, respiratory and bone infections, cystic fibrosis.

Adverse reactions: Thrombophlebitis, urticaria, pruritus, seizures, colitis.

Cautious use in renal impairment.

CARBAPENEM
Imipenem/Cilastatin

Dose: 60–100 mg/kg/day q6h IV. Maximum 4 g/day.

Indications: Drug of choice for ESBL. Aerobic and anaerobic microorganisms.

Adverse reactions: Diarrhea, vomiting, colitis, seizures.

Meropenem

Usual dose: 60 mg/kg/day q8h IV.

Meningitis: 40 mg/kg/dose q8h.

Neonatal sepsis: 20 mg/kg/dose q12h.

Indications: Drug of choice for extended spectrum beta lactamase producing microorganisms, also Streptococcus, *N. meningitidis* febrile neutropenia, respiratory tract infections.

Adverse reactions: Diarrhea, headache, vomiting, colitis, seizures, anaphylactic reactions.

Colistimethate

Dose: 50,000–75,000 IU/kg/day q8h IV.

Indications: Treatment of *Pseudomonas aeruginosa*, Enterobacter, Klebsiella.

Adverse reactions: Nephrotoxicity.

Colistin Sulphate

Dose: 5–15 mg/kg/day q6–8h oral.

Indications: Gram-negative bacillary diarrhea, bowel sensitization in neutropenic patients, *Pseudomonas enteritis.*

Contraindication: Myasthenia gravis.

Adverse reactions: Vomiting, diarrhea, neurotoxicity, nephrotoxicity.

Furazolidine

Dose: 6 mg/kg/day q6–8h oral.

Indications: Bacillary dysentery, giardiasis, food poisoning.

Adverse reactions: Orange-colored urine, nausea, headache, dizziness.

Contraindications: Infants <1 month, G6PD deficiency, primaquine sensitivity.

Linezolid

Dose: 20 mg/kg/day IV/oral q12h.

Indications: Treatment of vancomycin resistant enterococci and MRSA infections, community acquired and nosocomial pneumonia, febrile neutropenia.

Adverse reactions: Bone marrow depression, tongue discoloration, pseudomembranous colitis, lactic acidosis, seizures.

Caution: Protect from direct light, use suspension within 21 days after reconstitution, infuse over 30–120 minutes.

Nitrofurantoin

Usual dose: 5–7 mg/kg/day q6h oral with meals.

UTI prophylaxis: 1–2 mg/kg/day single oral dose at bedtime.

Indication: Treatment and prophylaxis of urinary tract infection.

Contraindications: Renal impairment, children <1 month, G6PD deficiency.

Adverse reactions: Fever, skin rash, hypersensitivity pneumonitis, liver toxicity.

Tigecyclin

Dose: 1.5 mg/kg single dose (maximum dose: 100 mg).

Maintenance: 1 mg/kg/day IV infusion over 30–60 min.

Indications: Gram-negative MDR, Acinetobacter ESBL, MRSA, carbepenam resistant *S. aureus*.

Adverse reaction: Hepatotoxicity.

Teicoplanin

Dose: 10 mg/kg/day BD for initial 3 doses, then 6–10 mg/kg/day OD IV/IM (bolus or slow IV infusion).

Indications: Gram-positive infections like MRSA and cephalosporin resistant *Staph. aureus*. Endocarditis prophylaxis, Gram-positive infections in neutropenic patients, pseudomembranous colitis.

Adverse reactions: Pain, phlebitis and abscess at injection site, rash, edema, vertigo, elevated liver enzymes.

Caution: Reduce the dose from day 4 in renal failure patients.

B. AGAINST GRAM-NEGATIVE ORGANISMS

AMPICILLIN (BETA LACTAM)

Dose: 100–200 mg/kg/day q4–6 hr IV/oral

For meningitis: 200–400 mg/kg/day q4 hr

For enteric fever: 200 mg/kg/day q6 hr oral

Indications: UTI, respiratory infection, meningitis, gonorrhea, typhoid, gastroenteritis, septicemia.

Contraindications: Infectious mononucleosis, hypersensitivity to penicillin.

Adverse reactions: Diarrhea, epigastric distress, rash.

Ceftriaxone (Cephalosporin 3rd Generation)

Dose: Usual dose of 50–75 mg/kg/day IV q12–24 hr in neonates, >2 g infants and children.

For meningitis: 100 mg/kg/day q12 hr IV.

Gonococcal ophthalmia neonatorum: 25–50 mg/kg/day IM/IV OD for 7 days.

N. meningitidis: 12 mg IM single dose to all contacts.

Typhoid: 50–100 mg/kg/day IM or IV 12–24 hrly.

Indications: Lower respiratory tract infection, bone and soft tissue infection, urinary tract infection, Salmonella gastroenteritis, typhoid, bacterial meningitis.

Contraindications: Hyperbilirubinemia, penicillin and cephalosporin hypersensitivity.

Adverse reactions: Pain after injection, diarrhea, hypersensitivity reaction, nephrotoxicity.

Do not use in neonates with hyperbilirubinemia, use cefotaxime instead as it displaces bilirubin from albumin binding site leading to increased free serum bilirubin levels.

Ciprofloxacin (Fluoroquinolones) 1st Generation

Dose: 20–40 mg/kg/day q12 hr oral OR 10–20 mg/kg/day 12 hr IV (maximum dose: 800 mg/day).

N. meningitidis contacts: 20 mg/kg single dose. IV is given over 30 minutes at 2 mg/ml.

Indications: UTI, gonorrhea, chancroid, bacterial gastroenteritis, typhoid, tuberculosis, meningitis

Caution: Renal disease and seizures.

Adverse reactions: GIT—nausea, vomiting, bad taste, CNS—dizziness, headache, restlessness, anxiety, skin rash, pruritus, photosensitivity.

Chloramphenicol (Broad Spectrum Antibiotic)
Dose:
Oral: 50–75 mg/kg/day q8 hr

iv: 100 mg/kg/day q6 hr

- <2 weeks of age: 25 mg/kg/day
- 2 weeks–1 yr: 50 mg/kg/day.

Indications: Enteric fever, *H. influenzae* meningitis, anaerobic infections.

Topical: Conjunctivitis, otitis externa.

Contraindications: Newborn <2 weeks, blood dyscrasias, porphyria, hypersensitivity.

Adverse reactions: Aplastic anemia, bone marrow suppression, gray baby syndrome.

Caution: G6PD deficiency

Gray baby syndrome occurs in newborn as chloramphenicol remains unmetabolised due to UDP-glucuronyl transferase enzyme deficiency (liver enzymes are not fully functional in newborn).

Azithromycin (Macrolide Antibiotic)

Dose:

- Usual dose: 10 mg/kg/day OD oral on empty stomach on day 1, followed by 5 mg/kg/day for next 4 days.
- Single dose of 30 mg/kg/day can also be given.
- Enteric fever: 20 mg/kg/day for 7–14 days.
- Cholera: 20 mg/kg single dose.

Indications: Otitis media, pharyngitis, tonsillitis, Gram-positive infections, endocarditis, enteric fever, cholera, cat-scratch disease, chlamydial infections.

Adverse reactions: Mild gastric upset, abdominal pain, headache, dizziness

Avoid in children <6 months.

Erythromycin

Dose:

Oral: 30–50 mg/kg/day in 4 divided doses for 14 days

iv: 5 mg/kg/dose infusion over 8 hr with normal saline or Ringer's lactate or intermittent bolus over 20–60 minutes q6–8 hr

Indications: Gram-positive infections, *Arcanobacterium haemolyticum,* feeding intolerance, chlamydial pneumonia, rheumatic fever prophylaxis, cholera, diphtheria, pertusis.

Contraindication: Liver diseases

Adverse reactions: Jaundice, epigastric pain, arrhythmias.

Clarithromycin

Dose: 15 mg/kg/day oral in 2 divided doses for 7 days

Indications: Respiratory tract and skin infections, sinusitis, otitis media, whooping cough, atypical pneumonia, *H. pylori* infections, leprosy.

Adverse reaction: Dyspepsia, anaphylaxis, Stevens-Johnson syndrome.

Doxycycline (Broad Spectrum Antibiotic)

Dose: 2–5 mg/kg/day BD oral.

Rickettsia: 2.2 mg/kg/dose q12 hr

Indications: Chronic bronchitis, brucellosis, Chlamydia, mycoplasma, rickettsia, cholera, acne.

Contraindication: Children <8 years of age.

Adverse reactions: Nausea, vomiting, diarrhea, phototoxicity, teeth staining.

AMINOGLYCOSIDE

Streptomycin

Dose: 15–20 mg/kg/day IM daily

Indications: Tuberculosis, endocarditis, plague, tularemia

Contraindications: Hypersensitivity, vestibular damage, myasthenia gravis.

Adverse reactions: Pain at injection site, ototoxicity, nephrotoxicity.

Amikacin

Dose: 15 mg/kg/day IM/IV q8–12 hr (maximum dose: 1 g).

Indications: Useful in atypical mycobacteria, septicemia, meningitis, bone, joint, CNS and lung infections, UTI, nosocomial infections.

Contraindication: Hypersensitivity.

Adverse reactions: Hearing loss, neuromuscular blockade, nephrotoxicity.

Netilmicin

Dose:
- ≤ 1 week: 3 mg/kg/dose q12 hr IV/IM
- >1 week: 2.5–3 mg/kg/dose q8h IV/IM

Infants: 7.5–10 mg/kg/day q8h IV/IM

Children: 6–7.5 mg/kg/day q8–12h IV/IM

Indications: Septicemia, renal, intra-abdominal, respiratory and genitourinary tract infections.

Adverse reactions: Nausea, hypersensitivity, ototoxic, nephrotoxic, neuromuscular blockade.

Tobramycin

More active against pseudomonas and proteus than gentamicin.

Dose: 6–7.5 mg/kg/day IV/IM q8–12h.

Indications: Neonatal septicemia, peritonitis, meningitis.

Adverse reactions: Skin rash, ototoxic, nephrotoxic.

Cotrimoxazole (Sulfamethoxazole-trimethoprim, ratio 5:1)

Dose:

Usual dose: 5–8 mg/kg of TMP or 25–50 mg/kg/day of SMZ q12 hr oral/IV.

Enteric fever: 10 mg/kg/day q12 hr of TMP

Pneumocystis carinii infection: 20 mg/kg/day q6–8 hr

Prophylaxis of Pneumocystis carinii: 5 mg/kg of TMP OD/ BD daily for 3 consecutive days in a week or alternate day.

UTI prophylaxis: 1–3 mg/kg/day of TMP single dose.

Indications: Urinary tract infection, respiratory tract infection, typhoid, bacterial diarrhea and dysentery.

Contraindications: Hypersensitivity to sulpha drugs, folate and G6PD deficiency, <6 weeks of age.

Adverse reactions: Stevens-Johnson syndrome, hepatic necrosis, agranulocytosis, megaloblastic anemia.

Nalidixic Acid

Dose: 50 mg/kg/day q6–8 hr oral.

UTI prophylaxis: 30 mg/kg/day q12 hr.

Indications: Use in diarrhea (caused by Proteus, *E. coli,* Shigella, Salmonella), and as urinary antiseptic.

Contraindications: Age <3 months, epilepsy, porphyrias.

Caution: Seizures, G6PD deficiency.

Adverse reactions: GIT upset, neurotoxicity, drowsiness, vertigo, raised ICT (pseudotumor cerebri), phototoxicity.

Aztreonam

Dose:

Children: 90–120 mg/kg/day q6–8h iv/im. iv bolus is given over 3–5 minutes or intermittent infusion over 20–60 min.

<7 days of age: 30 mg/kg/dose q8–12h.

Indications: Septicemia, urinary, lower respiratory and bone infections, Pseudomonas, Enterobacteriaceae.

Adverse reactions: Vomiting, diarrhea, rash, colitis, superinfections.

C. ANTITUBERCULAR DRUGS

1. FIRST LINE DRUGS

A. Isoniazid (H)

Dose: 5–10 mg/kg/day single dose oral on empty stomach. (Maximum dose: 300 mg)

Indication: First line antitubercular drug (multidrug therapy)

Contraindication: Hepatic damage

Adverse reactions: Hepatitis (rare), dizziness, seizures, peripheral neuritis, rash, fever.

B. Rifampicin (R)

Dose: 10–20 mg/kg/day single dose empty stomach

- Prophylaxis for *H. influenzae* type b: 20 mg/kg/day oral for 4 days.

- Prophylaxis for *N. meningitidis*
- Neonates: 10 mg/kg every 12 hr for 4 doses.
- >1 month: 20 mg/kg every 12 hr for 4 doses.

Indications: Leprosy, first line antitubercular drug, for brucellosis treatment along with doxycycline

CNS and genitourinary tuberculosis, prophylaxis of meningococcal and *H. influenzae* type b meningitis.

Contraindication: Hepatic damage

Adverse reactions: Hepatotoxicity, gastritis, orange-red urine, flu-like syndrome.

C. Pyrazinamide (Z)

Dose: 30–40 mg/kg/day single dose max up to 2 g

Indication as a component of MDT for tuberculosis

Contraindication: Hepatic damage, gout

Adverse reaction: Hepatotoxicity, arthralgia, hyperuricemia

D. Ethambutol (E)

Dose: 15–25 mg/kg/day single dose oral for 4 weeks and subsequently 15 mg/kg/day.

Indication: As a component of MDT for tuberculosis and MAC.

Adverse reaction: Optic and retrobulbar neuritis, hepatotoxicity.

Contraindication: Newborn, epilepsy, pre-existing optic neuritis.

E. Paraaminosalicylic Acid (PAS)

Dose: 200–400 mg/kg/day q8 hrly oral after food.

Indication: As a 2nd line drug for treatment of TB

Contraindication: Hypersensitivity

Adverse reactions: Hypokalemia, hepatitis, leucopenia, goiter

F. Ethionamide (Etm)

Dose: 15–20 mg/kg/day q12 hrly oral.

Indication: As 2nd line drug (in case of resistant TB)

Adverse reaction: Hepatotoxicity, peripheral neuropathy, tremor, optic neuritis.

Contraindications: Hypersensitivity, hepatic damage.

Use along with pyridoxine to prevent neurotoxicity.

G. Cycloserine (Cys)

Dose: 10 mg/kg/day q12 hrly orally

Indication: As a 2nd line bacteriostatic drug (in multidrug resistant TB)

Contraindication: Epilepsy, renal failure, depression.

Adverse reactions: Neurotoxicity, rash, megaloblastic anemia.

H. Kanamycin (Kmc)

Dose: 15 mg/kg/day 12–24 hourly IM.

Indication: As 2nd line drug for treatment of tuberculosis.

Wound and surgical site irrigation

Contraindication: Hypersensitivity

Adverse reactions: Nephrotoxicity, ototoxicity, pain at injection site.

I. Capreomycin (Cpr)

Dose: 15–30 mg/kg/day IM (maximum dose: 1 g)

Indication: Multidrug resistant tuberculosis.

Adverse reactions: Ototoxicity, nephrotoxicity, electrolyte abnormalities.

NEWER DRUGS

A. Ofloxacin

Dose: Oral: 15 mg/kg/day q12 hr.

IV: 5–10 mg/kg/day q12 hr.

Indications: *M. tuberculosis, M. avium* complex, *M. fortutium*

Leprosy, enteric fever, respiratory, GI and urinary infections, otitis externa, CSOM.

Contraindications: Hypersensitivity, convulsions.

Adverse reactions: GI upset, photosensitivity, arthralgia.

B. Clarithromycin

Dose: 15 mg/kg/day oral in 2 divided doses for 7 days

Indications: Respiratory tract and skin infections, sinusitis, otitis media, whooping cough, atypical pneumonia, *H. pylori* infections.

Adverse reactions: Dyspepsia, anaphylaxis, Stevens-Johnson syndrome.

C. Rifabutin

Dose:

- <6 years: 5 mg/kg/day q24 hrly orally
- >6 years: 300 mg/day OD

Indication: Multi-drug resistant tuberculosis

Prophylaxis and treatment of MAC (*Mycobacterium avium* complex)

Contraindication: Active tuberculosis, leucopenia, thrombocytopenia.

Adverse reactions: Red-orange urine, rash, dyspepsia.

D. ANTILEPROTIC DRUGS

Dapsone (DDS)

Dose: 1–2 mg/kg/day once daily (maximum: 100 mg/day).

Indications: Leprosy, dermatitis herpetiformis, prophylaxis against *Pneumocystis carinii* pneumonia.

Contraindication: G6PD deficiency

Adverse reactions: Hemolytic anemia, nephrotic syndrome, methemoglobinemia, agranulocytosis, peripheral neuropathy, SLE.

Clofazimine

Dose:

PO: 1 mg/kg/day OD daily (maximum dose: 50 mg/day) and 4–6 mg/kg maximum 300 mg once a month.

Lepra reaction: 100 mg twice or thrice daily for 21 days.

Indications: Multibacillary leprosy, chronic ulcers caused by *M. ulcerans*, lepra reaction.

Contraindications: peptic ulcer, diarrhea.

Adverse reactions: red discoloration of hair, urine, feces and other body secretions, phototoxicity, acneform eruptions.

Minocycline

Dose: Start with 4 mg/kg followed by 4 mg/kg/day q12 hr.

Indications: Veneral diseases, atypical pneumonia, cholera, brucellosis, plague, relapsing fever, rickettsial infections

Contraindication: Renal failure, children <8 years of age

Adverse reactions: Diarrhea, vestibular toxicity

4. Roxithromycin

Dose: 5–8 mg/kg/day BD oral

Indications: Sinusitis, pharyngitis, tonsillitis, acute bronchitis, pneumonia.

Adverse reactions: Nausea, skin rash, abdominal pain, diarrhea, oral candidiasis, flatulence.

Contraindications: Along with ergotamine alkaloids.

Advice: To be taken 30 minutes before food.

E. DRUGS FOR FUNGAL INFECTION

1. ANTIBIOTIC

A. Polyenes

a. Amphotericin B

Dose: 250 µg/kg/day increase to 1 mg/kg/day as IV infusion in 5% dextrose over 4–6 hr if interrupted for more than 7 days, then restart at 20 µg/kg/day.

Liposomal amphotericin B: 1–5 mg/kg/day

Amphotericin B lipid complex: 5–7 mg/kg/day.

Indications: Candidiasis, aspergillosis, blastomycosis, cocidiodomycosis, cryptococcosis, histoplasmosis, leishmaniasis, fungal endocarditis.

Adverse reactions: Fever with chills, vomiting, headache, hypomagnesemia, hypokalemia, azotemia.

Contraindications: Hepatic and renal disease.

b. Nystatin

Dose: 1–2 million units/day q4–6 hr oral.

Topical: Dissolve 100000 units nystatin per ml of glycerine.

Indications: Mucocutaneous, oral, vaginal, fungal infections.

c. Hamycin

Topical: Apply 2–3 times/day for 7–10 days.

Indications: Candidal oral thrush.

- Cutaneous candidiasis
- Monilial and trichomonas vaginitis
- Otomycosis by Aspergillus

B. Heterocyclic benzofurans

Griseofulvin

Dose: 5–15 mg/kg/day q6–12 hr oral, double dose in lesions involving nails of fingers and toes for 6–12 weeks.

Indications: Tinea infection of skin, hair and nails.

Adverse reactions: Headache, confusion, diarrhea, dizziness.

Contraindication: Porphyria. Candidial infection.

2. ANTIMETABOLITES

A. Flucytosine

Dose:

Neonates: 50–100 mg/kg/day q6 hr.

Children: 100–150 mg/kg/day q6–8 hr (maximum dose: 2 g/day).

Indication: Systemic yeast infections.

Adverse reactions: Bone marrow depression, neutropenia, thrombocytopenia, alopecia, hepatic and renal dysfunction.

3. AZOLES

A. Imidazoles (topical)

Clotrimazole

Topical: Apply twice or thrice daily.

Vaginal: Apply applicator full of 1% cream daily at bedtime for 7–10 days or 100–200 mg vaginal tablet for 3–7 days.

Indications: Oral and vaginal candidiasis, ringworm infections, superficial mycosis.

B. Triazoles (Systemic)

a. Fluconazole

Dose: 3–6 mg/kg/day once daily.

Invasive systemic candidiasis: 6–12 mg/kg/day for 28 days.

Indications: Candidiasis, cryptococcal meningitis, prophylactic agent for prevention.

Adverse reactions: Skin rash, abdominal pain, hepatic dysfunction, dizziness.

b. Itraconazole

Dose: 200–400 mg/day once daily orally for 12 weeks.

Indications: Aspergillosis, histioplasmosis, blastomycosis.

Adverse reactions: GI side effects, raised liver enzymes, hypokalemia.

c. Voriconazole

Dose: Start with 6 mg/kg q12 hr followed by 4 mg/kg q12 hr

Indications: Invasive aspergillosis, candidemia in non-neutropenic patients, fluconazole resistant serious Candida infections, Fusarium, Malassezia infections.

Adverse reactions: Skin rash, hepatotoxicity and photosensitivity.

d. Miconazole

Dose: PO

- <2 years: 2.5 ml twice daily
- 2–6 years: 5 ml twice daily
- >6 years: 5 ml 3 times a day
- Neonates: 5–15 mg/kg/day q8–24 hr
- IV dose is diluted with isotonic saline or 5% dextrose and given over 30–60 minutes.

Indications: Vulvovaginal candidiasis, topical treatment of superficial fungal infection.

Adverse reactions: Pruritis, skin rash, thrombocytopenia

Contraindications: Porphyria

e. Ketoconazole

Dose: 3.3 6.6 mg/kg/day once daily.

Indications: Systemic fungal infections, cutaneous dermatophytosis.

Contraindication: <2 years of age, liver disease

Adverse reactions: Suppression of testosterone synthesis and glucocorticoid secretion.

f. Terbinafine

Usual dose: 5–8 mg/kg/day single dose

- <20 kg: 62.5 mg oral single dose/day
- 20–40 kg: 125 mg/day single dose
- >40 kg: 250 mg/day single dose. For 2–12 weeks

Indications: Fungal infections of skin, hair and nails, onychomycosis.

Adverse reactions: Diarrhea, nausea, skin irritation, leucopenia.

g. Capsofungin

Dose: On day 1; 70 mg/m^2/day followed by 50 mg/m^2/day. Maximum: 70 mg/day.

Indications: Candidiasis, aspergillosis resistant or intolerant to amphotericin B, empirical therapy in febrile neutropenic patients.

Adverse reactions: Vomiting, nausea, dysphagia, thrombophlebitis and dystonia.

F. ANTIVIRAL DRUGS

1. Anti-herpes Virus

a. Idoxuridine

- Topical therapy for herpes simplex keratitis.
- Labila and gentila herpes

b. Acyclovir

Neonatal herpes: 10 mg/kg q8 hr IV for 14–21 days.

HSV encephalitis: 20 mg/kg q8 hr IV 21 days.

Varicella in immunocompetenthost: 80 mg/kg/day q6 hr for 5 days.

Herpes zoster: 800 mg q6 hr for 5 days.

Herpes simplex: 200 mg q4 hr for 5 days

Varicella zoster immunocompromised host: 80 mg/kg/d q8 hr

OR 250–600 mg/m^2/dose in 4–5 doses/day for 7–10 days.

Indications: Treatment of herpes zoster, herpes simplex encephalitis and keratitis, varicella in immunocompromised patients.

Contraindications: Liver and renal damage, epilepsy.

Adverse reactions: Phlebitis, extravasation, headache, rash, hypotension.

c. Famciclovir

Dose:

- Herpes zoster: 500 mg q for 7 days
- Genital herpes simplex: 250 mg q8 hr for 5 days
- Recurrent genital labialis: 1.5 g single dose
- Recurrent genital herpes: 250 mg BD for 1 year.

Indications: Against hepatitis B virus, herpes simplex, herpes zoster genital/labial herpes.

Adverse reactions: Hypotension, urinary retention, electrolyte imbalance.

d. Ganciclovir

Dose:

- Acquired CMV retinitis, pneumonitis, GI infections in immunocompromised host.
- Loading dose: 10 mg/kg/day q12 hr IV for 14–21 days. Maintenance dose: 5 mg/kg/day single daily dose.
- Prophylaxis of CMV in high-risk host: 10 mg/kg/day q12 hr IV for 7 days, then 5 mg/kg/day PO for 100 days.
- CMV peumonitis: 30 mg/kg/day q8 hr IV for 14 days.
- Oral: 30 mg/kg/dose q8 hr with food.

Indication: DOC for CMV infections

Congenital CMV pneumonia, acquired CMV retinitis in immunocompromised patients, HIV infection, prevention of CMV disease in transplant recipients, HSV1 and 2.

Adverse reactions: Hypertension, pancreatitis, neutropenia, electrolyte imbalance.

• Monitor platelets, blood counts, creatinine levels.
• Caution in bone marrow suppression.

e. Foscarnet

Dose: CMV retinitis in AIDS patients

Induction: 180 mg/kg/day q8 hr IV slow infusion over 1 hr for 21 days.

Maintenance: 90–120 mg/kg once daily.

Acyclovir resistant ASV and VZ in immunocompromised host: 120 mg/kg/day q8 hr IV till resolution of infection or 3 weeks.

Indications: Treatment of CMV, varicella zoster infections resistant to first line drugs, CMV retinitis.

Adverse reactions: Hypertension, seizures, dizziness, electrolyte imbalance.

Contraindication: Renal damage.

2. Anti-retro Virus

A. Nucleosidase Reverse Transcriptase Inhibitors (NRTIs)

a. Zidovudine (AZT)

Dose:

• Premature infants: IV—1.5 mg/kg; oral—2 mg/kg q8–12 hr
• <3 months: IV—1.5 mg/kg ; oral—2 mg/kg q8–12 hr

Pediatric dose: Oral: 90–180 mg/m^2 q6–8 hr.

Adult dose 200 mg QID initial, then 500–1500 mg/day 4–6 hr

Indications: symptomatic and asymptomatic HIV disease.

Chemoprophylaxis in HIV exposed individuals, prevention of vertical transmission of virus in pregnant woman.

Adverse reactions: Vomiting, abdominal pain, anemia, myalgia.

Contraindications: Bone marrow depression.

b. Didanosine

Dose:

Up to 90 days: 50 mg/m^2 q12 hr

Pediatric dose: 120 mg/m^2 q12 hr (maximum dose: 200 mg/dose)

Adolescent: Oral give 30 minutes before or 2 hr after meals.

- <60 kg—125 mg BD
- >60 kg—200 mg BD

Indications: In combination with other retroviral agents for treatment of HIV1 infections.

Adverse reactions: Pancreatitis, hepatomegaly, optic neuritis, peripheral neuropathy, anaphylactoid reaction.

c. Zalcitabine

Dose: Oral to be given 1 hr before or 2 hr after meals.

Pediatric dose: 0.01 mg/kg q8 hr

Adolescent dose: 0.75 mg/kg q8 hr

Adult dose: 1 mg q12 hr

Indications: Combination with other retroviral agents for treatment of HIV1 infections.

Adverse reactions: Peripheral neuropathy, fever, headache, leucopenia.

d. Stavudine

Dose: PO q12 hr
- <30 kg: 2 mg/kg/dose
- 30–60 kg: 30 mg/kg/dose
- >60 kg: 40 g/kg/dose

Adverse reactions: Headache, nausea, pancreatitis, peripheral neuropathy.

Avoid combination with Zidovudine

e. Lamivudine

Dose: PO

Neonates: 4 mg/kg/day q12 hr

Children: 4 mg/kg/dose q12 hr (maximum dose: 150 mg)

Adults: 300 mg OD

Indications: Management of HIV infection, chronic hepatitis B infection, postexposure prophylaxis.

Adverse reactions: Pancreatitis, paraesthesia, peripheral neuropathy, myalgia.

Contraindications: Renal damage

f. Abacavir

Dose: >3 months: 8 mg/kg q12 hr (maximum dose: 300 mg)

Adult dose: 300 mg BD/600 mg OD

Indications: Used as a second line drug.

Adverse reactions: Hypersensitivity reactions, vomiting, headache, rash.

B. Nonnucleosidase Reverse Transcriptase Inhibitors (NNRTIs)

Nevirapine

- Birth–6 weeks: <2 kg: 2 mg/kg or 0.2 ml/kg of suspension
- 2–2.5 kg: 10 mg OD or 1 ml OD of suspension
- >2.5 kg: 15 mg OD or 1.5 ml OD of suspension
- Neonates: 2 mg/kg single dose for prevention
- Children: 160–200 mg/m^2/dose oral BD.

Induction dose: Once daily for first 14 days, maintenance one-half of induction.

Adult: 200 mg OD for 2 weeks, increase the dose to 200 mg BD if no rash develops.

Indication: First line drug for prevention of vertical transmission as per NACO 2013 guidelines.

The duration of nevirapine prophylaxis is 6–12 weeks, if mother has not received ART prophylaxis from 24 weeks gestation.

Adverse reactions: Stevens-Johnson syndrome, skin rash, toxic epidermal necrolysis, liver dysfunction.

C. Protease Inhibitors

a. Ritonavir

Dose: PO given along with food.

Children: 400 mg/m^2/day BD increase by 50 mg/m^2/dose up to 800 mg/m^2/day BD

Adults: 400–600 mg/dose BD

Adverse reactions: Allergic reactions, photosensitivity, hepatitis, adrenocortical insufficiency

Contraindications: Not to give along with amiodarone, quinidine, midazolam.

b. Indinavir

Dose: 1.5 g/m²/day TDS.

Adverse reactions: Hyperglycemia, hyperlipidemia, nephrolithiasis.

c. Nelfinavir

Dose:
- <2 years: 30 mg/kg/day q8 hr
- >2 years: 50–55 mg/kg twice daily up to maximum of 2 g

Adult: 750 mg TDS.

Indication: Second line drug.

Adverse reactions: Diarrhea, nausea, rash.

d. Lopinavir in Combination with Ritonavir

Dose: Oral given along with food
- 7–15 kg: 12 mg/kg lopinavir + 3 mg/kg ritonavir q12 hr
- 15–40 kg: 10 mg/kg lopinavir + 2.5 mg/kg ritonavir q12 hr
- >12 years: 400 mg lopinavir + 100 mg ritonavir q12 hr

Indication: Against saquinavir and zidovudine resistant strains of HIV virus.

Used as a second line drug

Adverse reactions: Diarrhea, anemia, leucopenia, lymphadenopathy, DVT, Cushing's syndrome.

3. Anti-influenza Virus

a. Amantadine

Dose: 4–8 mg/kg/day q12–24 hr oral (maximum dose: <10 years–150 mg/day and >10 years–200 mg/day)

Duration of treatment until 24–48 hr after resolution of symptoms.

Adult dose: 200 mg OD/BD (maximum dose: 300 mg/day).

Indications: Prophylaxis and treatment of influenza A virus, herpes zoster, drug-induced extrapyramidal reactions, postencephalitis, parkinsonism.

Adverse reactions: Gout, arthralgia, confusion, urinary retention.

Contraindications: Epilepsy

b. Rimantadine

Prophylaxis and treatment of influenza A virus.

For prophylaxis: 1–9 years up to 40 kg: 5 mg/kg/day q12 hr (Maximum: 150 mg/day)

>10 years >40 kg: 100 mg BD

For treatment: 100 mg BD for 5–7 days.

Adverse reactions: Insomnia, nervousness, impaired concentration.

4. Non-selective Anti-viral Drugs

a. Ribavirin

Dose:

Aerosol inhalation: Dilute 6 g powder in 100 ml sterile water and nebulizer for 12–18 hr/day or 2 g over 2 hr 3 times daily for 3–7 days.

Oral: 10 mg/kg/day q6–8 hr (maximum dose: <10 years—150 mg/day and >10 years—200 mg/day)

Indications: Severe lower respiratory tract infection caused by respiratory syncytial virus, treatment of influenza A or B, adenovirus, chronic hepatitis C.

Adverse reactions: Dizziness, headache, pneumonia, cardiac arrest, apnea, anemia.

b. Adefovir dipivoxil

Dose: 10 mg/day oral given up to 5 years.

Indications: Chronic lamivudine resistant hepatitis B virus infection.

c. Interferon α

Dose:

- Chronic hepatitis B: 3–10 million units/m^2/day 3 times weekly.
- Chronic hepatitis C: 3 million units/m^2/day 3 times weekly.

Indications: Hepatitis B and C, AIDS related Kaposi's sarcoma, condyloma accuminata, malignant neoplasms.

Contraindications: Active tuberculosis, severe allergies, autoimmune hepatitis.

Adverse reactions: Flu-like symptoms, lethargy, neurotoxicity, myelosuppresion.

5. Miscellaneous
a. Adenine arabinoside

Dose: 15–30 mg/kg/day IV single dose during 12–24 hr for 10–21 days.

Indication: Herpes simplex infections.

b. Isoprinosine

Dose: 50–100 mg/kg/day q12 hr oral.

Indications: Viral encephalitis, subacute sclerosing panencephalitis (SSPE)

c. Oseltamivir

Dose:
- <3 months: 12 mg q12 hr; 3–5 months: 20 mg q12 hr; 6–11 months: 25 mg q12 hr for 5 days.
- <15 kg: 30 mg q12 hr; 15–23 kg: 45 mg q12 hr; 23–40 kg: 60 mg q12 hrs; >40 kg: 75 mg q12 hr oral for 5 days.

Prophylaxis: Once daily dosing for 7–10 days.

Indication: Treatment and prophylaxis of influenza A and B.

d. Valganciclovir

Indication and Dose
- Prophylaxis of CMV in post-transplant patient: 15–18 mg/kg/dose q6 hr oral for 100 days.
- CMV hepatitis, biliary atresia: 250 mg/m^2/day oral for 3 weeks.

e. Trifluridine

Dose: Topical 1 drop in each eye q2 hr (maximum dose: 9 drops). After re-epithelisation 1 drop every 4 hours (maximum dose: 5 drops).

Indication: Herpes simplex conjunctivitis and keratitis.

G. ANTIMALARIALS

A. 4-Aminoquinolines
Chloroquine
Chloroquine: 150 and 300 mg (base).

Dose: PO: Acute attack of malaria: Total dose 25 mg base/kg over 3 days, i.e. 10 mg base/kg stat, then 10 mg base/kg at 24 hr and 5 mg base/kg at 48 hr.

Prophylaxis: 5 mg base/kg once a week. Start 1 week before exposure and continue for 2–3 weeks after leaving endemic area.

Extraintestinal amoebiasis; PO—10 mg base/kg/day single dose for 2–3 weeks

(Maximum: 300 mg base/day).

Indications: DOC for prophylaxis of all types of malaria except that caused by resistant *P. falciparum*, extraintestinal amoebiasis, rheumatoid arthritis, discoid lupus erythematous, lepra reactions.

Contraindications: Liver damage, G6PD deficiency, seizure disorder, vision impairment.

Adverse reactions: Hypotension, cardiac depression, arrhythmias, CNS toxicity including convulsions.

Prolonged high dose (as in rheumatoid arthritis, DLE): Loss of vision due to Retinal damage.

B. Qulinoline-Methanol
Mefloquine
Dose: Treatment of drug resistant uncomplicated *P. falciparum* malaria; in combination with artesunate—25 mg/kg split over 2 days as 15 mg/kg and 10 mg/kg.

OR 8.3 mg/kg/day once a day for 3 days.

Prophylaxis: 3.5 mg/kg of base weekly.

Adult dose: Treatment—1250 mg single oral dose. Prophylaxis: 250 mg orally once a week for 4 weeks, then 250 mg every alternate week.

Indication: Treatment and prophylaxis of drug resistant/ chloroquine sensitive falciparum/vivax malaria.

Adverse reactions: Anxiety, neuropsychiatric reactions, hallucination, bradycardia, arrhythmias.

Contraindication: Renal impairment, seizure disorder, psychiatric illness, cardiac conduction defects.

C. Cinchona Alkaloids

a. Quinine

Quinine dihydrochloride

Loading dose: 20 mg/kg IV infusion slowly with 1 mg/ml of normal saline or 5% dextrose over 4 hr

Maintenance dose: 10 mg/kg/dose IV slowly over 4 hr q8 hr for 7–10 days.

Infusion rate not more than 5 mg salt/kg/hr.

Shift to oral therapy as soon as patient is taking orally.

IM route is as efficacious as IV. Loading dose 20 mg/kg diluted to 60 mg/ml divided and injected into both anterior and lateral aspects of thigh and bottocks followed by 10 mg/kg q8 hr.

Indications: Severe and complicated chloroquine resistant malaria

b. Quinine Sulfate

Dose: 30 mg/kg/day q8 hr oral for 7 days.

Used in combination with other drugs to prevent emergence of drug resistance.

Tetracycline: 40 mg/kg/day q6 hr for 10 days.

Clindamycin: 20–40 mg/kg/day q8 hr for 3 days.

Pyrimethamine: 0.75 mg/kg/day q12 hr for 3 days.

Sulfadiazine: 150 mg/kg/day q8 hr for 3 days.

Indication: Uncomplicated chloroquine resistant *P. falciparum* malaria.

Adverse reactions: Hypoglycemia, hypotension, cinchonism (prevented by giving with 5% dextrose).

Contraindications: Optic neuritis, myasthenia gravis, prolonged QT interval, G6PD deficiency, tinnitus, hemolytic anemia.

D. 8-Aminoquinoline
a. Primaquine

Dose: For radical cure: 0.25–0.5 mg base/kg/day oral OD for 14 days (maximum dose: 15 mg/day).

For falciparum: 0.7 mg/kg single dose.

Indication: Radical cure and prevention of relapse in *P. vivax* and ovale malaria and prophylaxis of *P. falciparum* malaria (destroys gametocytes).

Adverse reactions: Nausea, vomiting, hemolytic anemia, methemoglobinemia, leucopenia.

Contraindication: Rheumatoid arthritis, SLE, G6PD deficiency, children <1 year of age.

b. Pyrimethamine

Toxoplasmosis: 1 mg/kg/day oral q12 hr (maximum dose: 25 mg/day) for 3–6 weeks along with sulfadiazine 85 mg to 100 mg/kg/day q6 hr (maximum dose: 8 g/day).

If folic acid deficiency occurs, reduce the dosage or discontinue the drug and give leucovorin.

c. Pyrimethamine and Sulfadoxine

Dose:

Given along with artesunate.

Artesunate 4 mg/kg/day OD along with single administration of 20 mg or 1.0 mg/kg sulfadoxine–pyrimethamine on day 1.

Indication: Treatment of chloroquine resistant uncomplicated *P. falciparum* malaria.

Contraindications: Megaloblastic anemia, severe liver and renal impairment, infants <2 months of age, hypersensitivity to sulpha drugs.

Adverse reactions: Vomiting, unusual bleeding, rash, edema.

E. Tetracyclines
a. Tetracycline

Dose: 25–50 mg/kg/day q6 hr oral.

Indications: Respiratory, genitourinary and gastrointestinal infections, penicillin sensitive patients, aphthous ulcer, acne vulgaris, brucellosis.

Contraindication: Children <8 years, renal and liver impairment, SLE.

Adverse reactions: Hepatotoxicity, skin rash, discoloration of teeth, retardation of bone growth and teeth, thrombophlebitis, pseudotumor cerebri, pseudomembranous colitis and candidiasis.

b. Doxycycline

Dose: 2–5 mg/kg/day BD oral.

Rickettsia: 2.2 mg/kg/dose q12 hr

Indications: Chronic bronchitis, brucellosis, Chlamydia, mycoplasma, rickettsia, cholera, acne.

Contraindication: Children <8 years of age.

Adverse reactions: Nausea, vomiting, diarrhea, phototoxicity, teeth staining.

c. Artemether

Dose: 3.2 mg/kg IM on first day followed by 1.6 mg/kg daily for 5 days (total dose: 9.6 mg/kg).

Indications: Multidrug resistant and severe falciparum malaria including cerebral malaria with end organ damage.

Adverse reactions: Cardiotoxicity (QT prolongation, AV block), reduced reticulocytes and leucocytes, raised serum transaminases.

Contraindications: G6PD deficiency, immunocompromised patients.

d. Arteether

Dose: 3 mg/kg/day once daily for 3 days.

Indications: Severe and complicated falciparum malaria and cerebral malaria.

e. Lumefantrine

Available in fixed combination ratio of 1: 6. (artemeter plus lumefantrine)

- <3 years/5–14 kg: 1 tablet BD for 3 days
- 3–9 years/15–24 kg: 2 tablets BD for 3 days
- 9–14 years/25–34 kg: 3 tablets BD for 3 days
- >14 years/>34 kg: 4 tablets BD for 3 days

Indications: Treatment of falciparum malaria and new, recrudescent infection with a second course.

Adverse reactions: Headache, dizziness, myalgia, abdominal pain.

Contraindication: Cardiac patients.

F. Naphthoquinone

Atovaquone

Dose:
- <40 kg: 30–40 mg/kg/day oral once
- >40 kg: 750 mg/dose q8 hr oral for 21 days.

Indication: Alternative therapy for *Pneumocystis carinii* pneumonia in patients not tolerant to co-trimoxazole, babesiosis.

Adverse reactions: Diarrhea, vomiting, headache, rashes, fever.

H. ANTIAMOEBIC DRUGS

TISSUE AMOEBICIDE DRUGS

A. Nitroimidazoles

1. Metronidazole

Dose:

For amoebiasis (intestinal and extraintestinal): 35–50 mg/kg/day every 8 hr for 10 days.

For giardiasis: 15–20 mg/kg/day every 8 hr oral for 5–7 days.

For anaerobic infections: 20 mg/kg/day q6 hr oral/IV.

For antibiotic associated diarrhea: 20 mg/kg/dose q8 hr oral for 7–10 days (maximum dose: 400 mg/day).

Indications: Prevention and treatment of anaerobic infections, intra-abdominal infections and post-surgery, amoebiasis, giardiasis, trichomoniasis, ulcerative gingivitis, dental infections.

Contraindications: Hepatic failure, active CNS disease, blood dyscrasias.

Adverse reactions: Nausea, metallic taste, dry mouth, peripheral neuropathy, dark urine, seizures.

2. Tinidazole

For amoebiasis: 60 mg/kg/day single oral dose for 3 days.

For giardiasis: 50 mg/kg/day single oral dose.

Indications: Amoebiasis, giardiasis, ulcerative gingivitis, trichomoniasis, anaerobic infections.

Contraindications: Neurological disorders, blood dyscrasias.

Adverse reactions: Metallic taste, dark urine, neuropathy, seizures, leucopenia.

3. Secnidazole

Dose: 30 mg/kg single dose

For severe invasive diseases give for 5 days.

Indications: Amoebiasis, giardiasis.

Adverse reactions: Nausea, metallic taste, urticaria, cholestatic hepatitis.

4. Ornidazole

Dose:

Amoebiasis: 40 mg/kg OD for 3 days

Giardiasis: 40 mg/kg OD for 2 days

Indications: Giardiasis, amoebiasis, amoebic dysentery, anaerobic infections, trichomoniasis, bacterial vaginosis.

Adverse reactions: Nausea, abdominal pain, rash, headache.

B. Alkaloids

Dehydroemetine

Dose: 1.5 mg/kg/day IM for 10 days

If necessary, repeat the course 2 weeks later for another 10 days.

Indications: Amoebiasis, giardiasis, trichomoniasis

Adverse reactions: Cardiac and renal toxicity.

LUMINAL AMOEBICIDE DRUGS

A. Amide

Nitazoxanide

Dose: Oral q12 hr for 3 days.

1–3 years: 100 mg; 4–11 years: 200 mg; >12 years: 500 mg.

Indications: Giardiasis, cryptosporidiosis, *E. histolytica*, *Blastocystis hominis*, *Clostridium difficile*.

Adverse reactions: Dizziness, discolored urine, pale yellow eyes, increase in SGPT and serum creatinine.

B. 8-Hydroxyquinolines
Di-iodohydroxyquin
Dose: 30–40 mg/kg/day every 8 hr oral for 3 weeks.

Indication: Asymptomatic intestinal amoebiasis.

Contraindications: Hypersensitivity to iodine, liver damage.

C. Antibiotics
Tetracycline
Dose: 25–50 mg/kg/day q6 hr oral.

Indications: Respiratory, genitourinary and gastrointestinal infections, penicillin sensitive patients, aphthous ulcer, acne vulgaris, brucellosis.

Contraindications: Children <8 years, renal and liver impairment, SLE.

Adverse reactions: Hepatotoxicity, skin rash, discoloration of teeth, retardation of bone growth and teeth, thrombophlebitis, pseudotumor cerebri, pseudomembranous colitis and candidiasis.

I. ANTIHELMINTIC DRUGS

i. Mebendazole
Indications and Dose:
- For roundworm, hookworm and whipworm: 100 mg BD for 3 days
- For tapeworm and mixed infections: 200 mg BD for 3 days
- For pinworms: 100 mg single oral dose to be repeated after 2 weeks.
- For hydatid cyst 30 mg/kg/day every 8 hr for 4 weeks
- For trichinosis: 200 mg BD for 4 days.

Adverse reactions: Nausea, hair loss, granulocytopenia, expulsion of worm from mouth/nose.

Contraindication: Children <2 years

ii. Albendazole

Indications and Dose:

- Pinworms and roundworms: 1–2 years: 200 mg single dose oral
- >2 years: 400 mg single dose oral.
- Strongyloidosis, taeniasis and *H. nana*: 400 mg once daily for 3 days.
- Giardiasis: 400 mg daily for 5 days
- Hydatid disease: 400 mg twice daily for 28 days with fatty meals, may be repeated after 14 days interval for total of 3 cycles for eradication of hydatid disease.
- Neurocysticercosis: 15 mg/kg/day BD for 7 days along with corticosteroids for 5 days to reduce cerebral edema. Albendazole started on day 3 of steroid therapy.

Contraindications: Ocular and intraventricular cysticercosis, liver disease.

Adverse reactions: Nausea, dizziness, neutropenia.

iii. Pyrantel Pamoate

Indications and Dose:

- Ascaris, strongyloids, enterobius: 11 mg/kg single oral dose (maximum: 1g single dose).
- Ancylostoma: 10 mg/kg/dose oral OD for 3 days.

Contraindications: Hepatic disease, children <1 year, concurrent use of piperazine.

Adverse reactions: GIT symptoms, headache, dizziness, tenesmus.

iv. Piperazine

Indications and Dose:

- Roundworms: 75 mg/kg/day once daily for 2 days.
- For enterobius: 65 mg/kg/day once daily for 7 days.

Contraindication: Severe renal disease.

Adverse reactions: Nausea, abdominal pain, loss of coordination, dizziness.

v. Levamisole

Indications and Dose:

- Ascariasis: 2 mg/kg/day single oral dose.
- Ancylostomiasis: 2.5–5 mg/kg/dose or 50 mg q6 hr for 4 doses. Can be repeated after 7 days.
- Immunomodulator: 2 mg/kg/day 3 days in a week oral or alternate days for 4–6 weeks.

Contraindications: Liver and renal disease, psoriathric arthropathy.

Adverse reactions: Nausea, abdominal pain, insomnia, drowsiness.

vi. Diethylcarbamazine Citrate (DEC)

Dose:

- Filariasis: 6 mg/kg/day every 8 hr oral for 3–4 weeks.
- Tropical eosinophilia and visceral larva migrans: 10 mg/kg/day q8 hr oral for 1 month.
- Löffler's pneumonia: 15 mg/kg/day single dose for 4 days.

Adverse reactions: Nausea, anorexia, dizziness, headache.

vii. Ivermectin

Dose: 0.2 mg/kg single dose

Adult: 12 mg single dose. May repeat after 3–12 months.

Indications: Scabies, pediculosis, ascariasis, filariasis, onchocerciasis, strongyloidosis, visceral larva migrans.
Avoid below 5 years.

viii. Niclosamide

Dose: 1 g empty stomach followed by another dose after 1 hr. Give purgative after 2 hr of last dose. Give half the dose to <6 years of age. For *H. nana* single dose on day 1 and half the dose once a day for 6 days.

Indications: H. nana, D. latum, T. solium, T. saginata

Avoid below 2 years.

ix. Praziquantel

Indications and Dose:

- Neurocysticercosis: 50 mg/kg/day every 8 hr oral for 15 days with steroids

- Dermal cysticercosis: 60 mg/kg/day q8 hr for 6 days.
- *H. nana*: 25 mg/kg single oral dose.
- Tapeworms: 5–10 mg/kg single dose oral
- Schistosomiasis: 20 mg/kg/dose oral q8–12 hr for single day.
- Liverflukes: 75 mg/kg/dose q8 hr for 2 days.

Contraindication: Ocular and intraventricular cysticercosis.

Adverse reactions: Nausea, abdominal pain, itching, rashes, fever.

13

Anticancer Drugs

DRUGS ACTING DIRECTLY ON CELLS (CYTOTOXIC DRUGS)

A. ALKYLATING AGENTS

1. Nitrogen Mustards

a. Cyclophosphamide

Dose:

Minimal change nephrotic syndrome: PO; 2.5–3 mg/kg/day for 60–90 days when steroids are not successful.

SLE: 500–750 mg/m^2 IV every month. Maximum: 1g/m^2.

Preparatory regimen for bone marrow transplant: 50 mg/kg/day IV OD for 3–4 days.

For rest of the indications:

Start with 2–8 mg/kg/day oral followed by 2–5 mg/kg two times a week and IV: Start with 40–50 mg/kg in divided doses over 2–5 days followed by 10–15 mg/kg q7–10 days OR 3–5 mg/kg two times a week.

Indications: Treatment of germ cell ovarian tumors, disseminated neuroblastoma, Hodgkin's and non-Hodgkin's lymphoma, retinoblastoma, mycosis fungoides, SLE, nephrotic syndrome, multiple myeloma, leukemias. drug of choice for Wegener's granulomatosis.

Adverse reactions: Bone marrow depression, pancytopenia, hypoprothrombinemia, vomiting, alopecia, hemorrhagic cystitis.

Contraindications: Hypersensitivity.

144

b. Ifosfamide

Dose: IV; 1.2–1.8 g/m^2/day for 5 days q21–28 days or 5 g/m^2 as single 24 hr infusion or 3 g/m^2 day for 2 days.

Indications: Treatment of acute lymphoblastic leukemia, Hodgkin's lymphoma, Ewing sarcoma, breast, ovarian, testicular and lung cancers. Bronchogenic, breast, testicular, bladder, head and neck carcinomas, osteogenic sarcomas and some lymphomas.

Contraindication: Severely depressed bone marrow.

Adverse reactions: Hemorrhagic cystitis, hematuria, alopecia, vomiting, myelosuppression, pulmonary, liver, renal, CNS and cardiotoxicity.

c. Chlorambucil

Dose:

CML: Initially 0.4 mg/kg increase by 0.1 mg/kg q2 weeks single daily dose until myelosuppression occurs.

For rest of indications: 0.1–0.2 mg/kg/day (Avg: 4–10 mg/day) daily for 3–6 weeks, then 0.03–0.1 mg/kg/day (Avg: 2–4 mg/day) for maintenance.

Indications: Palliative treatment for advanced Hodgkin's disease, non-Hodgkin's lymphoma, nephrotic syndrome, polycythemia vera, CLL.

Adverse reactions: Bone marrow depression, GI side effects, rash.

2. Ethylenimine

Thio-TEPA

Dose: 25–65 mg/m^2 IV as a single dose q3–4 weeks.

Indications: Treatment of adenocarcinoma of breast and ovary, Hodgkin's disease, lymphomas, sarcoma.

Adverse reactions: Pain at injection site, headache, dizziness, pancytopenia, bone marrow depression.

Contraindications: Severe myelosuppression.

3. Alkyl sulfonate

Busulfan

Dose: 0.06–0.12 mg/kg oral once daily.

Indications: Chronic myeloid leukemia, acute myelocytic leukemia.

Adverse reactions: Stomatitis, vomiting, headache, bone marrow depression and seizures, hyperuricemia, pulmonary fibrosis, adrenal insufficiency.

4. Triazine

Dacarbazine (DTIC)

Indications and Dose:

Neuroblastoma: 800–900 mg/m^2 single IV dose every 3–4 weeks.

Solid tumors: 200–470 mg/m^2/day IV over 5 days every 21–28 days.

Hodgkin disease: 375 mg/m^2 on day 1 and day 15; repeat every 28 days.

Indication: Neuroblastoma, soft tissue sarcoma.

Adverse reactions: Nausea, vomiting, anorexia, blood dyscrasias, bone marrow depression.

B. ANTIMETABOLITES

1. Folate Antagonist

Methotrexate (Mtx)

Dose: Juvenile rheumatoid arthritis: 5–15 mg/m^2/week single dose or 3 divided doses 12 hr apart.

Antineoplastic dose: 7.5–30 mg/m^2/week oral/IM.

Indications: Juvenile rheumatoid arthritis and other autoimmune diseases.

Choriocarcinoma, acute leukemias, non-Hodgkin's lymphoma, osteogenic sarcoma and other solid tumors.

Contraindications: Bone marrow suppression, renal and hepatic impairment.

Adverse reactions: Megaloblastic anemia, pancytopenia, mucositis, diarrhea, desquamation and bleeding from GIT.

2. Purine Antagonist

a. 6-mercaptopurine (6-MP)

Dose: 2.5–5 mg/kg/day once daily oral followed by half the dose for maintenance.

Indication: Acute lymphoblastic leukemia.

Contraindications: Liver disease, severe bone marrow suppression.

Adverse reactions: Myelosuppression, liver necrosis, gastroenteritis.

b. Azathioprine

Kidney transplant: Initial dose: 2–5 mg/kg/day

Maintenance dose: 1–3 mg/kg/day oral once a day.

For rheumatoid arthritis and SLE: 1 mg/kg/day. Maximum dose 2.5 mg/kg/day for 6–8 weeks.

Indications:

- Prevention of renal and other graft rejections
- Rheumatoid arthritis, SLE, steroid resistant nephritic syndrome, inflammatory bowel disease

Adverse reactions: Bone marrow depression, liver damage, leucopenia, thrombocytopenia, skin cancers, intestinal ulcers, hyperurecemia.

c. Fludarabine

Indication and Dose:

- Acute leukemia: 10 mg/m^2 IV bolus over 15 minutes followed by continuous infusion of 30.5 mg/m^2/day over 5 days.
- Solid tumors: 9 mg/m^2 bolus followed by 27 mg/m^2/day for 5 days.

Adverse reactions: Fever, vomiting, pneumonia, bone marrow toxicity, tumor lysis syndrome.

3. Pyrimidine Antagonist

a. 5-fluorouracil (5-FU)

Loading dose of 12 mg/kg/day IV for 4–5 days (maximum dose: 800 mg/day).

Maintenance dose: 6 mg/kg IV daily for 4 doses; repeat in 4 weeks.

Colorectal carcinoma/hepatoma: 15–20 mg/kg/day for 5–8 days or 15 mg/kg/wk.

Indications: Treatment of carcinoma of breast, colon, stomach, hepatoma, superficial basal cell carcinoma.

Adverse reactions: Stomatitis, pruritic rash, pancytopenia, agranulocytosis.

Contraindications: Bone marrow depression, surgery within 1 month, poor nutritional status.

b. Cytarabine (cytosine arabinoside)

Leukemia, non-Hodgkin lymphoma: 70–200 mg/m^2/day IV for 2–5 days each month.

OR 1–1.5 mg/m single IM/SC dose at 1–4 weeks interval.

Indications: Treatment and induction of remission in acute lymphocytic leukemia, AML, CML, meningeal leukemia, non-Hodgkin lymphoma.

Adverse reaction: Asthenia, fever, change in taste, bone marrow depression.

C. VINCA ALKALOIDS

1. Vincristine (oncovin)

Dose: 1–2 mg/m^2 IV. Maximum dose: 2 mg.

Indications: Treatment of acute leukemia, neuroblastoma, rhabdomyosarcoma, Wilms' tumor, non-Hodgkin lymphoma.

Adverse reactions: Peripheral neuropathy, paresthesia, alopecia, bronchospasm, foot/wrist drop.

2. Vinblastine

Dose: 2.5–6 mg/m^2/day OD IV every 1–2 weeks for 3–6 weeks (maximum dose: 12.5 mg/m^2)

For germ cell tumor: 0.2 mg/kg on day 1 and day 2 every 3 weeks for 4 cycles.

Indications: Treatment of germ cell tumor, histiocytosis, non-Hodgkin lymphoma, choriocarcinoma, neuroblastoma, CML, advance stage of mycosis fungoides.

Adverse reactions: Vomiting, alopecia, leucopenia, liver toxicity.

Contraindications: Bacterial infections, granulocytopenia.

D. TAXANES

Paclitaxel

Dose: 250–350 mg/m^2/dose by IV infusion over 24 hrs, repeated every 3 weeks.

Indication: Metastatic ovarian and breast carcinoma after failure of 1st line chemotherapy and relapse cases, Wilms' tumor.

Adverse reactions: Reversible myelosupression, stocking and glove neuropathy, chest pain, arthralgia, myalgia, mucositis, edema, acute anaphylactoid reaction due to camphor solvent.

E. EPIPODOPHYLLOTOXIN
Etoposide

Dose: 60–150 mg/m^2/ day IV or oral for 2–5 days every 3–6 weeks.

Indication: Treatment of AML, AIDS associated Kaposi sarcoma, Ewing sarcoma.

Adverse reactions: Alopecia, vomiting, bone marrow depression, leucopenia, GI disturbances.

F. ANTIBIOTICS
1. Doxorubicin

Dose: 35–75 mg/m^2 IV q3 weeks.

Indications: Treatment of Wilms' tumor, soft tissue and bone sarcomas, Hodgkin and non-Hodgkins lymphoma, regression in ALL and AML.

Contraindications: Cardiomyopathy, myelosuppression, congestive cardiac failure.

Adverse reactions: Vomiting, alopecia, bone marrow depression, cardiotoxicity.

2. Daunorubicin (rubidomycin)

Dose: AML; 30–60 mg/m^2 IV daily for 3 days, repeat weekly

ALL: 25–45 mg/m^2 on days 1 and 8 of cycle.

Indication: Acute leukemia

Adverse reactions: Cardiotoxicity, marrow depression, alopecia, stomatitis, vomiting.

Contraindications: Arrhythmia, cardiac failure, bone marrow suppression.

3. Mitoxantrone

Dose: 12 mg/m² once daily for 2–3 days.

Indications: Acute non-lymphocytic leukemia, acute leukemia in relapse, solid tumors, non-Hodgkin's lymphoma.

Adverse reactions: Bone marrow depression, renal failure, sepsis, pneumonia.

Contraindications: Cardiac failure, liver impairment.

4. Mitomycin C

Dose: 10–20 mg/m² single IV dose; repeat q6–8 hr

Indications: Treatment of disseminated adenocarcinoma of pancreas and stomach, CML.

Adverse reactions: Bone marrow depression, renal and pulmonary toxicity, vomiting, fever, anorexia.

Contraindications: Coagulation disorders and bleeding tendency.

Monitor WBC and platelet counts.

G. MISCELLANEOUS

1. Hydroxyurea

Dose: 10–20 mg/kg once daily.

Sickle cell anemia: 15 mg/kg once daily.

Indications: Resistant chronic myelocytic leukemia, sickle cell anemia, polycythemia vera

Adverse reaction: Myelosuppression

Contraindication: TLC count <2500 and platelet <1 lac.

2. Procarbazine

Dose: 100–200 mg/m²/day once daily oral.

Indications: Treatment of advanced Hodgkin's disease, neuroblastoma, aplastic anemia, polycythemia vera, brain tumors.

Adverse reactions: Vomiting, stomatitis, myalgia, bone marrow depression, UTI, arthralgia.

3. L-asparginase

Dose: 1000 units/kg/day for 10 days (combination therapy). 200 units/kg/day for 28 days (single drug therapy).

Indications: Leukemias, Hodgkin's disease, melanosarcoma.

Adverse reactions: Liver damage, allergic reactions like urticaria, arthralgia, pancreatitis.

4. Cisplatin

Dose: 15–20 mg/m^2/day for 5 days IV every 3–4 weeks.

Indications: Metastatic testicular and ovarian cancer, osteogenic sarcoma, neuroblastoma, brain tumor, bone marrow/stem cell transplant.

Adverse reactions: Vomiting, nephrotoxicity, tinnitus, deafness, neuropathy, hyperurecemia, anaphylactic reaction.

Contraindications: Hearing and renal impairment, myelo-suppression.

5. Carboplatin

Dose:
- Solid tumor: 560 mg/m^2 q4 weeks
- Brain tumor: 175 mg/m^2 q4 weeks
- Sarcoma: 400 mg/m^2/day for 2 days

Indications: Bony and soft tissue sarcoma, germ cell tumors, pediatric brain tumor, bone marrow transplant preparation.

Contraindication: Bone marrow depression, allergic reactions, severe bleeding.

Adverse reactions: Peripheral neurotoxicity, bone marrow suppression.

6. Imatinib

Dose: 260 mg/m^2 single dose or 2 divided doses oral.

Indication: Chronic myeloid leukemia.

Adverse reactions: Fluid retention, edema, vomiting, abdominal pain, myalgia, neutropenia.

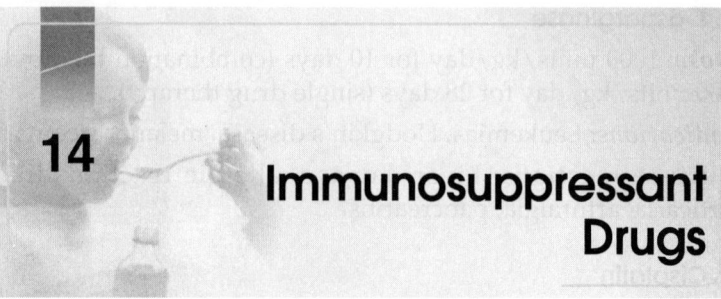

14 Immunosuppressant Drugs

CALCINEURIN INHIBITORS

1. Cyclosporin

Dose: Prevention of allograft rejection: 10–15 mg/kg/day with milk or fruit juice, gradually reduce to 2–6 mg/kg/day as maintenance for 6 months to 1 year.

IV dose is 1/3rd of oral dose (5–6 mg/kg) slowly over 2–6 hr.

Indications:

- Prevention of graft rejection in organ transplant.
- Autoimmune diseases, alopecia, corneal transplant, aplastic anemia.

Adverse reactions: Nephrotoxicity, hepatotoxicity, hypertension, hyperkalemia, hyperurecemia, opportunistic infections, hirsutism, tremor.

2. Tacrolimus

Dose:

- Oral: 0.2 mg/kg BD
- Topically: 0.03% 2 times a day.

Indications: Prophylaxis of organ transplant rejection, autoimmune diseases, atopic dermatitis.

Contraindication: Simultaneous use with cyclosporine.

Adverse reactions: Nephrotoxicity, pleural effusion, thrombo-cytopenia, neurotoxicity.

m-TOR INHIBITORS

Sirolimus

Dose: Loading dose 3 mg/m² daily, followed by 1 mg/m²/day maintenance dose.

Indication: Prophylaxis of organ transplant rejection.

Adverse reactions: Thrombocytopenia, hypercholesterolemia, diarrhea, hypertension.

ANTIPROLIFERATIVE DRUGS

1. Azathioprine

Dose:

- Kidney transplant: Initial dose: 2–5 mg/kg/day
- Maintenance dose: 1–3 mg/kg/day oral once a day.
- For rheumatoid arthritis and SLE: 1 mg/kg/day. Maximum dose 2.5 mg/kg/day for 6–8 weeks.

Indications:

- Prevention of renal and other graft rejections
- Rheumatoid arthritis, SLE, steroid resistant nephritic syndrome, inflammatory bowel disease

Adverse reactions: Bone marrow depression, liver damage, leucopenia, thrombocytopenia, skin cancers, intestinal ulcers, hyperurecemia.

2. Methotrexate

Dose:

- Juvenile rheumatoid arthritis: 5–15 mg/m²/week single dose or 3 divided doses 12 hr apart.
- Antineoplastic dose: 7.5–30 mg/m²/week oral/IM.

Indications:

- Juvenile rheumatoid arthritis and other autoimmune diseases
- Choriocarcinoma, acute leukemias, non-Hodgkin's lymphoma, osteogenic sarcoma.

Contraindications: Bone marrow suppression, renal and hepatic impairment.

Adverse reactions: Megaloblastic anemia, pancytopenia, mucositis, diarrhea, desquamation and bleeding from GIT.

3. Cyclophosphamide

Minimal change nephrotic syndrome: PO; 2.5–3 mg/kg/day for 60–90 days when steroids are not successful.

SLE: 500–750 mg/m² IV every month. Maximum: 1g/m².

Preparatory regimen for bone marrow transplant: 50 mg/kg/day IV OD for 3–4 days.

For rest of the indications:

Start with 2–8 mg/kg/day oral followed by 2–5 mg/kg two times a week and

IV: Start with 40–50 mg/kg in divided doses over 2–5 days followed by 10–15 mg/kg q7–10 days OR 3–5 mg/kg two times a week.

Indications: Treatment of germ cell ovarian tumors, disseminated neuroblastoma, Hodgkin's and non-Hodgkin's lymphoma, retinoblastoma, mycosis fungoides, SLE, nephrotic syndrome, multiple myeloma, leukemias.

Adverse reactions: Bone marrow depression, pancytopenia, hypoprothrombinemia, vomiting, alopecia.

4. Chlorambucil

Dose:

CML: Initially 0.4 mg/kg increase by 0.1 mg/kg q2 weeks single daily dose until myelosuppression occurs.

For rest of indications: 0.1–0.2 mg/kg/day (Avg: 4–10 mg/day) daily for 3–6 weeks, then 0.03–0.1 mg/kg/day (Avg: 2–4 mg/day) for maintenance.

Indications: Palliative treatment for advanced Hodgkin's disease, non-Hodgkin's lymphoma,

Nephrotic syndrome, polycythemia vera.

Adverse reactions: Bone marrow depression, GI side effects, rash.

GLUCOCORTICOIDS

Prednisolone

Four times more potent than hydrocortisone.

Dose: 1–2 mg/kg/day q6–8 hr oral after meals.

Indications: All inflammatory disease conditions, allergic conditions, asthma, rheumatic fever, nephrotic syndrome, autoimmune disease, malignancy, pemphigus.

Contraindications: Systemic infection, peptic ulcer, live virus immunization, herpes simplex keratitis.

Adverse reactions: Increased chances of infection, edema, hypertension, hyperglycemia, psychosis, Cushing syndrome

BIOLOGICAL AGENTS
A. TNF-α Inhibitors
Etanercept

Dose: 4–17 years; 0.4 mg/kg/dose sc twice weekly given 3–4 days apart (maximum dose: 25 mg).

Indications: Rheumatoid arthritis, Crohn's disease.

Contraindication: Serious active infection.

Adverse reactions: Pain at injection site, pyelonephritis, pneumonia, bronchitis, cellulitis.

B. IL-2 Receptor Antagonist
1. Daclizumab

Dose: 1 mg/kg IV over 15 minutes. First dose is given 24 hr before transplantation and then 14 days later. Total 5 doses. (maximum dose: 100 mg).

Indications: Prophylaxis of renal and other transplant rejection reaction, graft vs host disease.

Adverse reactions: Headache, arthralgia, vomiting.

2. Basiliximab

Dose:
- >35 kg: 2 doses of 20 mg each in reconstituted volume of 50 ml given as IV infusion over 20–30 minutes.
- 20 mg is given 2 hr before transplant and second dose of 20 mg 4 days after transplant.
- <35 kg: 10 mg.

Indications: Prophylaxis of renal and other transplant rejection reaction.

Adverse reactions: Constipation, headache, respiratory infection, dysuria.

C. Anti-CD3 Antibody
1. Muromonab CD3
Dose:
- <12 years: 0.1 mg/kg/day for 10–14 days.
- >12 years: 5 mg/day for 10–14 days.

Indication: Treatment of acute allograft rejection.

Adverse reactions: Cytokine release syndrome, pulmonary edema, seizure, shock-like state.

Contraindications: Fluid overload, >3% weight gain.

D. Polyclonal Antibodies
Rho (D) immunoglobulin
Indications and Dose:

For idiopathic thrombocytopenic purpura

Loading dose: 50 μg/kg single dose IV.

Maintenance dose: 25–60 μg/kg based on platelet and Hb levels.

Abortion, miscarriage, termination of ectopic pregnancy:
- <13 weeks of gestation: 300 μg IM.
- >13 weeks of gestation: 50 μg IM.

Contraindication: IgA deficiency.

Adverse reactions: Hypotension, pallor, vasodilation.

DYES
1. Gentian violet
Dose: 0.5–1% aqueous or alcoholic solution

Indication: Mucocutaneous and cutaneous infection caused by *Candida albicans*.

2. Triple dye
Acriflavine 1.14 g, gentian violet 2.29 g, brilliant green 2.29 g and distilled water or spirit 1L for topical application.

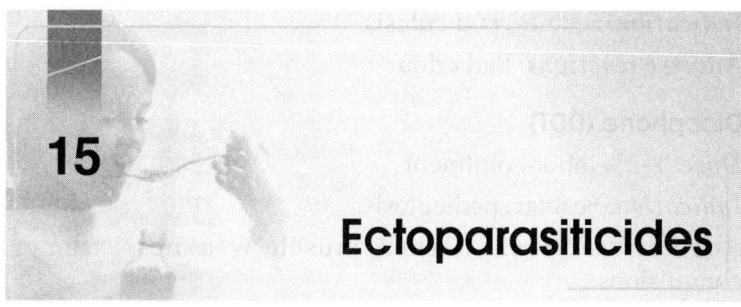

15

Ectoparasiticides

Permethrin (5% cream)

- At night after bath apply from head to toe. Apply twice in a whole week treat simultaneously all contacts.
- Pediculosis: Shampoo the hair and towel dry, apply 1% lotion over scalp and rinse after 10 minutes. Repeat after 1 week and treat all contacts.

Indications: Scabies, pediculosis.

Adverse reactions: Mild and transient burning, itching, tingling, erythema, rash

Lindane (BHC)

Dose: 1% lotion, ointment

Indications: Lice, mites, scabies.

Adverse reactions: CNS stimulation, vertigo, convulsions, cardiac arrhythmias.

Benzyl benzoate

Dose: 25% lotion, ointment

Indication: Scabies

Contraindication: Children who have neurological symptoms

Adverse reactions: Skin irritation, contact dermatitis.

Sulfur

Dose: 10% ointment

Indication: Scabies, pediculosis
Adverse reactions: Bad odour

Dicophane (DDT)
Dose: 1–2% lotion, ointment
Indication: Scabies, pediculosis.
Adverse reactions: Rashes, muscle weakness, tremor, convulsions.

Ivermectin
Dose: 0.2 mg/kg single dose
Adult: 12 mg single dose. May repeat after 3–12 months.
Indications: Scabies, pediculosis, ascariasis, filariasis, onchocerciasis, strongyloidosis, visceral larva migrans.
Avoid below 5 years.

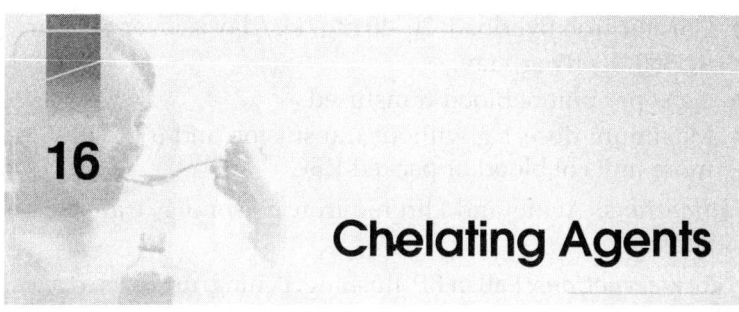

16

Chelating Agents

DIMERCAPROL (BAL)

Dose: 2.5–4 mg/kg/dose q4–6 hr for 2 days followed by 2.5 mg/kg dose q12 hr for 10 days.

Indications: Poisoning by arsenic, mercury, gold, bismuth, nickel, platinum, as adjuvant to calcium disodium edetate in lead poisoning as adjuvant to penicillamine in copper poisoning and Wilson's disease.

Contraindication: Iron and cadmium poisoning.

PENICILLAMINE

Dose: 20–40 mg/kg/day oral q6–8 hr empty stomach.

Up to 10 years: 0.5–0.75 g/day; >10 years: 1 g/day q12 hr before meals.

Add vitamin B_6 and zinc.

Indication: Wilson disease, heavy metal poisoning, cystinuria, rheumatoid arthritis.

Adverse reactions: Cutaneous reaction, itching, febrile episodes, dermatological, renal, hematological and collagen toxicities.

DESFERRIOXAMINE

- Acute iron intoxication: 1 g is given stat followed by 500 mg every 4 hr for 2 days, then 500 mg q4–12 hr depending on the response. Maximum dose: 6 g/day.
- Intravenous infusion rate should not be more than 15 mg/kg/hr for the first 1 g, subsequently 125 mg/hr.

- Chronic iron overload: 20–40 mg/kg/day sc over 8–12 hr
- IM: 500–1000 mg/day.
- 2 g IV per unit of blood transfused.
- Maximum dose 1 g without transfusion and 6 g with 3 or more units of blood or packed RBC.

Indications: Acute and chronic iron poisoning, transfusion siderosis.

Adverse reactions: Fall in BP, flushing, itching, urticaria, rashes, allergic reactions.

Contraindication: Acute renal failure.

DEFERIPRONE

Dose: 50–100 mg/kg daily q6–12 hr oral.

Indication: Transfusion siderosis in hemolytic anemia, thalassemia.

Adverse reactions: Anorexia, vomiting, altered taste, joint pain, reversible neutropenia, agranulocytosis.

Deferasirox

Indication: Iron overload due to chronic hemolytic anemia and repeated blood transfusion.

Dose: 20–35 mg/kg single oral dose on empty stomach.

- Dose is titrated to maintain serum ferritin level below 500 mg/ml.
- Not recommended for below 2 years of age.

17

Vitamins

VITAMIN A

- Fat soluble vitamin
- Daily requirement: 400–1000 IU/day. 1 IU = 0.3 µg retinol

Dose:

Vitamin A deficiency with xerophthalmia: Oral—same dose is repeated after 4 weeks.

- <6 months: 50,000 IU
- 6–12 months: 1,00,000 IU
- >12 months: 2,00,000 IU

For prophylaxis of patients at risk and supplementation with measles vaccine; <1 year: 1 lac IU; >1 year: 2 lac IU oral every 6 months.

Prevention of bronchopulmonary dysplasia: 5000 IU im 3 days in a week for 28 days.

Improvement of growth:

- <1 year: 1 lac IU for 2 doses, then at 4 and 8 months.
- >1 year: 2 lac IU for 2 doses, then at 4 and 8 months.

Indications: Vitamin A prophylaxis, xerophthalmia, night blindness, psoriasis, prevention of BPD in neonates, improvement of growth in AIDS and malaria.

Contraindication: Hypervitaminosis A.

Adverse reactions: Fatigue, irritability, mental changes, anorexia, stomach discomfort.

VITAMIN B

i. Vitamin B$_1$ (Thiamine)

Daily requirement: 0.1–1 mg or 0.5 mg/1000 kcal diet

Dose:

- Beriberi: IM/IV 10–25 mg/day; oral: 10–50 mg/day for 2 weeks, then 5–10 mg/day for 1 month.
- Metabolic disease: 100 mg q8 hr.

Indications: Treatment of beriberi and Wernicke's encephalopathy, peripheral neuritis, anorexia nervosa.

Adverse reactions: Cardiovascular collapse, angioedema, rash, tingling.

ii. Vitamin B$_2$ (Riboflavin)

Daily requirement: 0.1–2 mg or 0.6 mg/1000 kcal diet.

For deficiency: 2.5–10 mg/day q8–12 hr

For metabolic disease: 50–150 mg q12–24 hr

iii. Vitamin B$_6$ (Pyridoxine)

Daily requirement: 0.1–0.6 mg/day

Dose:

- For deficiency: 5–15 mg/day for 3–4 weeks then 2.5–5 mg/day.
- Prevention of isoniazid neuropathy: 10 mg/day and for treatment 50 mg q8 hr oral.

Indications: Pyridoxine seizures in newborn, prophylaxis and treatment of vitamin B$_6$ deficiency, sideroblastic anemia.

Adverse reactions: Nausea, decreased serum folic acid, seizures.

iv. B$_{12}$ (Cyanocobalamin)

Dose

- Premature: 200 µg PO
- Full term: 40 µg PO
- Premature: 0.4 mg PO
- Full term: 0.6 mg PO

- Premature: 400 µg PO
- Full term: 35 µg PO
- Premature: 1.5 µg PO
- Full term: 0.15 µg PO

Indications

- Treatment and prevention of thiamine deficiency, including a specific disorder called Wernicke-Korsakoff syndrome (WKS).
- Preventing and treating riboflavin deficiency and conditions related to riboflavin deficiency.
- Treatment and prevention of pyridoxine deficiency.
- Treating a type of anemia called sideroblastic anemia.
- Treating some types of seizures in infants when given intravenously
- Treatment and prevention of vitamin B_{12} deficiency, and diseases caused by low vitamin B_{12} levels.
- Treatment of pernicious anemia.

Contraindications

- Serious hypersensitivity reaction.
- It can occur after IV and IM dose signs of an allergic reaction
- Long-term use of high doses is POSSIBLY UNSAFE. It might cause certain brain and nerve problems.
- Pregnancy and breastfeeding.
- The treatment of vitamin B_{12} deficiency can unmask the symptoms of polycythemia vera.
- Leber's disease, a hereditary eye disease: Do not take vitamin B_{12} if you have this disease. It can seriously harm the optic nerve, which might lead to blindness.

Side effects

- Feeling of warmth, pruritis, nausea, pulmonary edema.
- Yellow discoloration of urine in large doses
- Sensory neuropathy, ataxia.
- Perioral numbness
- Asthenia, weakness
- Glossitis

VITAMIN C

Dose: 1.25 mg equivalent to 50,000 USP units

Indications

- Vitamin/mineral supplementation
- Hypoparathyroidism
- Osteomalacia
- Renal osteodystrophy
- Rickets
- Familial hypophosphatemia
- Vitamin D deficiency

Contraindication: No contraindications.

Side effects: Polyuria, nocturia, polydipsia, hypercalciuria, reversible azotemia, hypertension, nephrocalcinosis, generalized vascular calcification, irreversible renal insufficiency (may be fatal), mental retardation, widespread soft tissue calcification, osteoporosis, dwarfism, vague aches, stiffness, weakness, nausea, anorexia, constipation, mild acidosis, anemia, weight loss.

VITAMIN D

Dose: Infants 0–6 months, 2 µg; infants 6–12 months, 2.5 µg; children 1–3 years, 30 µg; children 4–8 years, 55 µg; children 9–13 years, 60 µg.

Indications:

- Treating and preventing vitamin K deficiency. Vitamin K_1 can prevent and treat vitamin K deficiency.
- Preventing certain bleeding or blood clotting problems. Vitamin K_1 can prevent bleeding or blood clotting problems in newborns.
- Reversing the effects of too much warfarin used to prevent blood clotting. Taking vitamin K_1 can counteract too much anticoagulation caused by warfarin.

Contraindications:

- Liver disease
- Kidney disease

Side effects:

- Anaphylactoid reaction

- Hyperbilirubinemia
- Vitamin B$_{12}$ (cyanocobalamin)

Daily requirement: 0.3–2 μg/day.

Therapeutic dose: 250–1000 μg IM on alternate day for 1–2 weeks, then weekly until blood count is normal.

Maintenance dose: 1000 μg 2–4 months.

Indications: Treatment of vitamin B$_{12}$ glossitis, pernicious anemia.

Adverse reactions: Hypersensitivity reaction on injection, anaphylactoid reaction.

VITAMIN C (ASCORBIC ACID)

Daily requirement: 30 mg/day in term babies.

Preterm: 50 mg/day

Older children: 40 mg/day

Therapeutic dose: 100–300 mg/day oral/IV OD.

Indications: Treatment of scurvy, to enhance iron absorption along with ferrous salts in anemia, methemoglobinemia.

Adverse reactions: GI upset, renal stones.

VITAMIN E (TOCOPHEROL)

Neonates: 6–12 IU/kg/day oral (maximum dose: 25–50 IU/day).

Children: 1 IU/kg/day

Sickle cell anemia: 450 IU/day

Beta thalassemia: 750 IU/day

Cystic fibrosis: 100–400 IU/day

Indications: Prevention of anemia of prematurity, broncho-pulmonary dysplasia, Rett syndrome, treatment of vitamin E deficiency, nocturnal muscle cramps, as an antioxidant.

Adverse reactions: Nausea, weakness, fatigue, abdominal cramps.

FOLIC ACID

Physiological requirements:

Newborn: 25–35 μg/day

Up to 3 years: 50 µg/day

4–6 years: 75 µg/day

7–10 years: 100 µg/day

11–14 years: 150 µg/day

Therapeutic dose: 2–5 µg/day

Prophylactic dose: 0.5 µg/day

Indications: Megaloblastic anemia, hemolytic anemia, severe iron deficiency anemia, celiac disease, tropical sprue, along with phenytoin.

Folic acid should always be given along with vitamin B_{12} in patients with vitamin B_{12} deficiency.

No adverse effects.

Alfacalcidol (1-alphahydroxycholecalciferol)

A prodrug that is rapidly hydroxylated in liver to calcitriol so does not require hydroxylation in kidney.

Premature infants: 0.1 µg/kg/day

<20 kg: 0.05 µg/kg/day oral

>20 kg: 1 µg/kg/day oral.

Renal osteodystrophy: 0.04–0.08 µg/kg/day.

Indications: Renal osteodystrophy, vitamin D dependent and resistant rickets, hypoparathyroidism, osteomalacia.

Contraindications: Hyperphosphataemia, hypercalcaemia, vitamin D toxicity.

18

Drugs and Specific Dosages in Newborn

ACYCLOVIR

Dose:

- Neonatal herpes: 10 mg/kg q8 hr IV for 14–21 days.
- HSV encephalitis: 20 mg/kg q8 hr IV 21 days.
- Varicella in immunocompetent host: 80 mg/kg/day q6 hr for 5 days.
- Herpes zoster: 800 mg q6 hr for 5 days.
- Herpes simplex: 200 mg q4 hr for 5 days
- Varicella zoster immunocompromised host: 80 mg/kg/d q8 hr

OR 250–600 mg/m^2/dose in 4–5 doses/day for 7–10 days.

Indications: Treatment of herpes zoster, herpes simplex encephalitis and keratitis, varicella in immunocompromised patients.

Contraindications: Liver and renal damage, epilepsy.

Adverse reactions: Phlebitis, extravasation, headache, rash, hypotension.

ALBUMIN

Dose:

- Hypoproteinemia: 0.5–1 g/kg/dose IV. Repeat every 1–2 days.
- Rate of administration should not exceed 2 ml/min over 2–4 hr.

- Hypovolemia: 0.5–1 g/kg/dose. Maximum dose: 6 g/kg/day. Rapid infusion.
- Cerebral edema: 50–80 ml/kg rapid infusion.

Indications: Burns, hypovolemia, hypoproteinemia, plasma volume expansion and maintenance of cardiac output, prior to exchange transfusion in neonatal jaundice, cerebral edema, nephrotic syndrome.

Contraindications: Congestive heart failure, severe anemia, pulmonary edema.

Adverse reactions: Fluid overload, congestive heart failure.

Albumin 5% used for hypovolemia and 25% for patients with fluid or sodium restriction.

AMPICILLIN

Postnatal age ≤7 days
- <2 kg: 50 mg/kg/day IM/IV q12 hr; Meningitis: 100 mg/kg/day IV/IM BD
- >2 kg: 75 mg/kg/day IV/IM q8 hr; Meningitis: 150 mg/kg/day IV/IM q8 hr

Postnatal age >7 days
- <1.2 kg: 50 mg/kg/day IV/IM q12 hr; Meningitis: 100 mg/kg/day IV/IM q12 hr
- 1.2–2 kg: 75 mg/kg/day IV/IM q8 hr; Meningitis: 150 mg/kg/day IV/IM q8 hr
- >2 kg: 100 mg/kg/day IV/IM q6 hr; Meningitis: 200 mg/kg/day IV/IM q6 hr

CEFOTAXIME SODIUM
- ≤ 7 days: 100 mg/kg/day IV/IM q12 hr
- >7 days: <1.2 kg–100 mg/kg/day IV/IM q12 hr
- >1.2 kg: 150 mg/kg/day IV/IM q12 hr

CEFTAZIDIME
- Postnatal age ≤7 days: 100 mg/kg/day IV/IM q12 hr.
- Postnatal age >7 days:
- <1.2 kg: 100 mg/kg/day IV/IM q12 hr >1.2 kg: 150 mg/kg/day IV/IM q12 hr.

CEFTRIAXONE SODIUM

- Systemic infections: 50 mg/kg/day IV/IM OD
- Meningitis: 100 mg/kg/day IV/IM OD.

ENOXAPARIN

Dose: SC

- <2 months prophylaxis: 0.75 mg/kg/dose q12 hr. Treatment: 1–5 mg/kg/d q12 hr.
- >2 months–<18 months prophylaxis: 0.5 mg/kg/dose q12 hr. Treatment: 1 mg/kg/dose q12 hr.

Indications: DIC, purpura fulminans, prophylaxis and treatment of thromboembolism.

Contraindications: Bleeding disorder, GI ulcer.

Overdose treated with protamine sulfate.

EPINEPHRINE

- Severe bradycardia and hypotension
- IV push: 0.1–0.3 ml/kg of 1:10000 concentration (equal to 0.01–0.03 mg/kg or 10–30 µg/kg)
- May repeat 3–5 min up to 3–4 times.
- Continuous infusion: Start at 0.1 µg/kg/min. Maximum dose: 1 µg/kg/min.

ERYTHROMYCIN

Dose: PO

- Postnatal age ≤7 days: q12h—20 mg/kg/day.
- Postnatal age >7 days >2 kg: q6–8 h—30 mg/kg/day
- <1.2 kg: q12h—20 mg/kg/day.
- Fluconazole dosing interval for invasive candidiasis
- Oral thrush; On day 1: 6 mg/kg/day IV/oral OD
- Then 3 mg/kg/day OD for 14–21 days.
- Systemic infections: Postnatal age <14 days: 6–12 mg/kg/day IV/oral every 72 hr
- >14 days: 6–12 mg/kg/day IV/oral OD.

GENTAMICIN SULFATE

- Postnatal age <7 days: IV/IM
- 1.2–2 kg: 2.5 mg/kg/dose q12–18 hr; >2 kg: 2.5 mg/kg/dose BD.
- Postnatal age >7 days: IV/IM.
- 1.2–2 kg: 2.5 mg/kg/dose q8–12 hr; > 2 kg: 2.5 mg/kg/dose TDS.

HYDROCORTISONE

- Adrenal insufficiency: 1–2 mg/kg/dose IV bolus, then 25–150 mg/day q6 hr–q8 hr.
- Congenital adrenal hyperplasia: 0.5–0.7 mg/kg/day IV, then 0.3–0.4 mg/kg/day. Give quarter in morning and afternoon and half at night.

INDOMETHACIN

For closure of patent ductus arteriosus: 0.1–0.25 mg/kg/dose IV BD for 3–6 doses.

SURFACTANTS

Beractant (survanta)

- Prophylactic: 4 ml/kg/dose intratracheally as soon as possible.
- Bovine lung surfactant divided into 4 aliquots, with up to 3 additional doses (4 total), administered q6h if needed during the first 48 hr.
- Rescue therapy: 4 ml/kg/dose intratracheally immediately following the diagnosis of RDS. May repeat 4 doses as needed q6 hr.

Calfactant (infasurf)

Dose: 3 ml/kg/dose

Bovine lung surfactant divided into 2 aliquots, with up to 2 additional doses administered q12h if needed.

Poractant alfa (corosurf)

- Initial dose = 2.5 ml/kg/dose. Subsequent dose = 1.25 ml/kg/dose

- Porcine lung surfactant divided into 2 aliquots, followed by up to 2 additional doses of 1.25 ml/kg/dose, administered.
- Method of administration:
- Prior to administration suction infant with 5 F feeding tube. Each dose is divided into 41 ml/kg aliquots; administer 1 ml/kg in each of four different positions over 2–3 sec.

Adverse reactions: Pallor, bradycardia, hypotension, apnea, pulmonary air leak.

VANCOMYCIN
Postnatal age ≤7 days
- <1.2 kg: 15 mg/kg/dose IV q24h
- 1.2–2 kg: 10–15 mg/kg/dose IV q12–18h
- >2 kg: 30 mg/kg/dose IV q12h

Postnatal age: > 7 days
- <1.2 kg: 15 mg/kg/dose IV q24h
- 1.2–2 kg: 10–15 mg/kg/dose IV q8–12h
- >2 kg: 45 mg/kg/dose IV q8h

ZIDOVUDINE
Preterm infant: ≤ 2 weeks: 1.5 mg/kg/dose oral q12h

> 2 weeks: 2 mg/kg/dose oral q8h

Term infant: 8 mg/kg/day oral q6 hr OR 6 mg/kg/day IV q6h

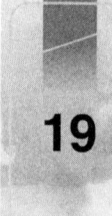

19   Vaccines and Immunoglobulins

BCG

Content: 0.1 to 0.4 million viable bovine mycobacteria

Nature and diluents: Lyophilized, normal saline

Storage: Freezer/2 to 8°C

Protect from light

Dose: 0.1 ml ID

Site: Left deltoid

Schedule: Single dose at birth or first contact below 5 years

Efficacy: 0–80%

Adverse reactions: Axillary lymphadenitis

Contraindications: Cellular immunodeficiency should not be given with measles/MMR.

OPV

Content: Sabin strain

Nature: Liquid vaccine

Storage: Freezer/2 to 8°C

Dose: 2 drops oral

Schedule: Birth, 6, 10, 14 weeks, 15–18 months, 5 years, NID, SNID

Efficacy: 10–15% per dose (India), 30% per dose (world)

Adverse reactions: Rarely VAPP

Contraindication: Immunodeficient patients and household contacts.

IPV

Content: Salk strain

Nature: Liquid vaccine

Storage: 2 to 8°C

Dose and route: 0.5 ml IM or SC, thigh deltoid

Schedule: 6, 10, 14 weeks, booster at 15–18 months

Efficacy: 95–100%

Adverse reactions: None

Contraindication: Serious hypersensitivity

DTwP/DTaP

Content: Diphtheria toxoid 20–30 Lf, tetanus toxoid 5–25 Lf, wP 4 IU/aP 3 µg to 25 µg of 2 to 5 purified pertussis antigens

Nature: Liquid vaccine

Storage: 2 to 8°C. Protect DTaP from light.

Dose and route: 0.5 ml IM thigh/deltoid

Schedule: 6, 10, 14 weeks, booster at 15–18 months, 5 years

Not recommended above 7 years

Efficacy: 95–100% for diphtheria/tetanus and 70–90% for pertussis

Adverse reactions: Rare. More with DTwP. High fever, excessive crying, seizures, HHE, encephalopathy.

Contraindications: Serious hypersensitivity, encephalopathy following previous dose.

TT

Content: Tetanus toxoid 5 Lf

Nature: Liquid vaccine

Storage: 2 to 8°C

Dose and route: 0.5 ml IM thigh/deltoid

Schedule: As routine at 10 years and every 10 years thereafter, pregnancy, wound management (Td/Tdap preferred to TT)

Measles

Content: 1000 CCID50 of Edmonston Zagreb strain of measles virus

Nature: Lyophilized, diluent sterile water

Storage: Freezer/2 to 8°C
Protect from light

Dose and route: 0.5 ml sc thigh/deltoid

Schedule: Single dose at 9 months

Efficacy: 80%

Adverse reactions: Mild measles like illness in <5%. Rarely thrombocytopenic purpura.

Contraindications: Severely immunocompromised, pregnancy

Rubella

Content: 5000 CCID50 of RA27/3 strain of rubella virus

Nature: Lyophilized, diluent sterile water

Storage: Freezer/2 to 8°C

Dose and route: 0.5 ml sc thigh/deltoid
As for MMR, MMR preferred.

Efficacy: 95%

Adverse reactions: Mild rubella like illness in <5%, rarely arthritis, ITP

Contraindications: Severely immunocompromised, pregnancy.

MMR

Content: Measles and rubella as above Mumps 5000 CCID of 50 Jeryl Lynn/Urabe strain

Nature: Lyophilized, diluent sterile water

Storage: Freezer/2 to 8°C
Protect from light

Dose and route: 0.5 ml sc thigh/deltoid

Schedule: Two doses at 15–18 months and 5 years

Efficacy: 95%

Adverse reactions: Same as measles and rubella, high fever, rarely parotid swelling, aseptic meningitis

Contraindications: Severely immuno-compromised, pregnancy

Hep B

Content: 20 µg/ml of HBsAg antigen

Nature: Liquid vaccine

Storage: 2 to 8°C

Dose and route: <18 years: 0.5 ml, >18 years: 1 ml IM deltoid/thigh

Schedule: Birth, 6, 14 weeks OR 6, 10, 14 weeks OR 0, 1, 6 months

Efficacy: >90%

Adverse reactions: None

Contraindication: Serious hypersensitivity

Hib

Content: 10 µg of PRP-T or HbOC

Nature: Liquid or lyophilized (diluent sterile water)

Storage: 2 to 8°C

Dose and route: 0.5 ml IM deltoid/thigh

Schedule: 6, 10, 14 weeks, booster at 15–18 months

Efficacy: >90%

Adverse reaction: None

Contraindication: Serious hypersensitivity

Vi typhoid

Content: 25–30 µg of Vi polysaccharide

Nature: Liquid vaccine

Storage: 2 to 8°C

Dose and route: 0.5 ml IM deltoid/thigh

Schedule: Above 2 years, single dose, revaccination every 3 years

Efficacy: 60%

Adverse reactions: None

Contraindication: Serious hypersensitivity

HPV

Content: Quadrivalent L1 protein of serotypes 6, 11, 16, 18
Nature: Liquid vaccine
Storage: 2 to 8°C. Protect from light.
Dose and route: 0.5 ml IM deltoid
Schedule: 10–12 years, 0, 2, 6 months
Efficacy: >95% against serotype-specific cervical cancer
Adverse reactions: None
Contraindications: Serious hypersensitivity, pregnancy.

HPV

Nature: Bivalent L1 protein of serotypes 16, 18
Schedule: 10–12 years 0, 1, 6 months

PCV

Content: Capsular polysaccharide of serotypes 4, 6B, 9V, 14, 18C, 19F, 23,1, 5, 6A, 19A, 7F, 3 linked to CRM 197
Nature: Liquid vaccine
Storage: 2 to 8°C
Dose and route: 0.5 ml IM thigh/deltoid
Schedule: 6, 10, 14 weeks, booster at 15–18 months
Efficacy: 95% against serotype-specific invasive disease
Adverse reaction: None
Contraindieation: Serious hypersensitivity

PPV23

Content: Capsular polysaccharides of 23 serotypes
Nature: Liquid vaccine
Storage: 2 to 8°C
Dose and route: 0.5 ml SC/IM thigh/deltoid
Schedule: Single dose at >2 years. Revaccination only once after 3–5 years.
Efficacy: 70% against invasive disease in high-risk children
Adverse reactions: None
Contraindication: Serious hypersensitivity

Inactivated Hep A

Content: HM 175 strain composition varies with brands/age

Nature: Liquid vaccine

Storage: 2 to 8°C

Below 15/18 years (as per brand)

Dose and route: 0.5 ml IM deltoid/thigh

Schedule: Two doses 6 months apart, 18 months onwards

Efficacy: >95%

Adverse reactions: None

Contraindication: Serious hypersensitivity

Hep A and Hep B

Content: Composition varies with age

Nature: Liquid vaccine

Storage: 2 to 8°C

Below 18 years

Dose: 0.5 ml

Schedule: 0, 1 and 6 months, 18 months onwards

Efficacy: >95%

Adverse reactions: None

Contraindication: Serious hypersensitivity

Live attenuated Hep A

Content: 6.5 log particles of H_2 strain

Nature: Lyophilized, sterile water

Storage: 2 to 8°C

Dose and route: 1 ml SC deltoid/thigh

Schedule: Two doses 6 months apart 18 months onwards till 15 years.

Efficacy: >95%

Adverse reactions: None

Contraindication: Immunodeficient patients

Varicella

Content: >1000 PFU of Oka strain

Nature: Lyophilized, sterile water

Storage: 2 to 8°C. Protect from light.

Dose and route: 0.5 ml sc deltoid/thigh

Schedule: <13 years 2 doses, at 16 months and 5 years

　　　　　　>13 years two doses 4–8 weeks apart

Efficacy: 70–90% with one dose, >95% with 2 doses

Adverse reactions: Varicella like rash in 5%

Contraindication: Pregnancy, severely immunocompromised

Rotavirus (monovalent) LAV

Content: Human rotavirus strain 89–12 (G1P8)

Nature: Lyophilized, sterile water-based specific liquid diluent

Storage: 2 to 8°C. Protect from light.

Dose and route: 1 ml orally

Schedule: 2 doses, first dose at 6–15 weeks, second at least 4 weeks later. Schedule to be completed by 32 weeks and not to be initiated after 15 weeks.

Efficacy: 85–98% against severe rotavirus diarrhea

Adverse reactions: None

Contraindication: Acute gastroenteritis, beyond 6 months

Human Bovine Pentavalent vaccine

Content: 5 rotavirus reassortant strains G1, G2, G3, G and P1A[8]

Nature: Liquid vaccine

Storage: 2 to 80

Dose and route: 2 ml orally

Schedule: 3 doses,1st dose at 6–15 weeks and then at 4 weeks interval schedule to be completed by 32 weeks.

Efficacy: 85–98% against severe rotavirus diarrhea

Adverse reaction: None

Contraindication: Beyond 32 weeks age

Inactivated influenza

Content: Split virus vaccine having 7.5–15 µg of three chosen strains

Nature: Liquid vaccine

Storage: 2 to 8°C

Dose and route: 0.25 ml for 6 months to 3 years and 0.5 ml for older children IM deltoid/thigh

Schedule: First time: <9 years two doses 1 month apart, >9 years single dose. Revaccination: annually

Efficacy: 50–90% against lab confirmed disease

Adverse reactions: None

Contraindication: Severe egg allergy, history of GBS

Rabies

Content: Inactivated rabies virus grown on human diploid/ chick embryo or vero cells

Nature: Lyophilized, diluent sterile water

Storage: 2 to 8°C

Dose and route: 1 ml (0.5 ml for vero cell vaccine), IM deltoid/thigh

Schedule: Any age 0, 3, 7, 14 and 28 days for post-exposure and 0, 7 and 28 days for pre-exposure

Efficacy: 90–100% (along with RIG, if indicated)

Inactivated JE vaccine

Content: Nakayama/Beijing strain of JE virus

Nature: Lyophilized, diluent sterile water

Storage: 2 to 8°C

Dose and route: 0.5 ml for 1–3 years and 1 ml for >3 years SC deltoid

Schedule: Three doses at 0, 7 and 30 days, boosters every 2–3 years

Efficacy: 80–90%

Adverse reactions: Rarely allergic reactions/acute neurologic events

Contraindication: Serious hypersensitivity

Live JE vaccine

Content: 5.4 log PFU of SA 14-14-2 strain of JE virus

Nature: Liquid vaccine

Storage: 2 to 8°C

Dose and route: 0.5 ml SC thigh/deltoid

Schedule: Single dose at >9 months

Efficacy: >90%

Adverse reactions: None

Contraindication: Immunodeficient patients and their household contacts

MPSV

Content: Bivalent (A + C) Quadrivalent (A + C + Y + W135)

Nature: Lyophilized, diluent sterile water

Storage: 2 to 8°C

Dose and route: 0.5 ml SC or IM thigh/deltoid

Schedule: If indicated, single dose above 2 years, revaccination once after 3–5 years.

Efficacy: 90%

Adverse reactions: None

Contraindication: Serious hypersensitivity

Yellow Fever (LAV)

Content: 17 D strain of yellow fever virus

Nature: Lyophilized/saline diluents

Storage: 2 to 8°C

Dose and route: 0.5 ml SC thigh/deltoid

Schedule: Single dose, revaccination every 10 years, if needed

Efficacy: >90%

Adverse reactions: Rarely neurologic/viscerotropic disease

Contraindications: Below 6 months, serious egg allergy, severe immune-deficiency, thymus disease

Cholera

Nature: Liquid vaccine

Storage: 2 to 8°C

Dose and route: 1.5 ml oral

Schedule: Two doses above 1 year and 6 weeks apart

Efficacy: 60%

20

Poisons and Antidotes

1. Acetaminophen (Paracetamol)

N-acetyl cysteine
- Initially 140 mg/kg then 70 mg/kg 4 hr for additional 17 doses via nasogastric tube/orally. Repeat dose if vomiting occurs within 1 hr of administration.
- IV: Loading dose: 150 mg/kg in 5% dextrose over 15 minutes.
- Maintenance dose: 50 mg/kg in 5% dextrose q6–8 hr for 3 doses.

2. Anticholinergics (Atropine, Belladona)

Physostigmine 0.02 mg/kg/dose or 0.5 mg IV/SC/IM every 5 minutes till desired effect is reached (maximum dose: 2 g).

3. Amphetamine (Toxic dose: 50 mg)

Chlorpromazine 1 mg/kg IM/IV (maximum dose: IV dose 50 mg).

4. Benzodiazepine

Flumazenil IV in incremental dose of 0.1, 0.2, 0.3 and 0.5 mg at 1 minute interval until desired effect is reached.

5. Carbon monoxide

100% oxygen till carboxyhemoglobin level is <10%.

6. Cyanide (Fatal dose)

Amyl nitrate, inhalation for 15–30 sec of each minute, then sodium nitrate 3% solution, 0.2–0.4 ml/kg IV at rate of

2.5–5 ml/min (maximum dose: 10 ml) followed by sodium thiosulfate 1–2 ml/kg (maximum dose: 50 ml) of 25% solution over 10 min. Use lower doses, i.e. 0.2 ml/kg for children with anemia.

Adverse reactions: Methemoglobinemia.

7. Ethylene Glycol

• Ethanol 10 ml/kg 10% solution iv or 1 ml/kg of 95% solution by mouth.
• Maintenance dose: 1.5 ml/kg/hr 10% solution iv or 3 ml/kg/hr 10% solution iv during hemodialysis.

8. Mercury

• British Anti-Lewisite (BAL)
  – Day 1 and 2, 3–5 mg/kg im every 4 hr; day 3 and 4: 2.5–3 mg/kg q6 hr
  – After 1 week: 2.5–3 mg/kg q12 hr course can be repeated after 5 days.

9. Arsenic

• British Anti-Lewisite (BAL)
  – Day 1 and 2: 3–5 mg/kg im q4 hr; Day 3 and 4: 2.5–3 mg/kg q6 hr
  – After 1 week: 2.5–3 mg/kg q12 hr. Course can be repeated after 5 days.

10. Lead

• British Anti-Lewisite (BAL):
  – Day 1 and 2: 3–5 mg/kg im every 4 hours; Day 3 and 4: 2.5–3 mg/kg q6 hr
  – After 1 week: 2.5–3 mg/kg q12 hr. Course can be repeated after 5 days.
    Calcium disodium ethylene diamine tetraacetic acid (EDTA): 50–75 mg/kg/day in 4 divided doses im/iv as 0.2–0.4% solution.
  – For symptomatic children (blood level >70 µg/dl in asymptomatic children): Dimercaprol 75 mg/m² im q4 hr (total daily dose: 450 mg/m²) followed by EDTA 1.5 g/

m^2/day by continuous infusion for 5 days. BAL is stopped when lead levels are <60 µg/dl. Repeated courses may be needed till blood levels are <20 µg/dl.

- For asymptomatic children (levels: 45–69 µg/dl): EDTA $1g/m^2$/day infusion for 5 days.
- d-penicillamine 20–40 mg/kg/day q6–8 hr empty stomach orally for 5 days.
- Oral thiamine and dimercaptosuccinic acid (DMSA) 350 mg/m^2/dose q8 hr oral for 5 days, then every 12 hr for 14 days. Give supplements of calcium and iron.

11. Heparin

Protamine sulfate: 2.5–5 mg/kg IV followed by 1–2.5 mg/kg IV q4 hr (1 mg protamine is used for 100 units of heparin as 1% solution IV).

12. Iron

- Desferrioxamine: 15 mg/kg/hr IV infusion (maximum dose: 6 g/day)
- Therapy needed for 12–36 hr till urine color becomes normal
OR
- 90 mg/kg/dose IM q8 hr

13. Isoniazid

- Pyridoxine: 1 mg IV to be given for each 1 mg of isoniazid.
- If amount of isoniazid ingested is not known, then give 500 mg pyridoxine IV over 30 minutes.

14. Warfarin

Vitamin K: 5–10 mg IV/IM, repeat every 6–8 hr

15. Propranolol

Glucagon: 50–150 µg/kg bolus followed by 50 µg/kg/hr infusion.

16. Methylalcohol

- Ethanol: loading dose: 10 ml/kg of 10% solution of ethanol IV.
- Maintenance: 1.5 ml/kg/hr infusion.

- Oral: 1 ml/kg of 95% ethanol in fruit juice over 30 min and then 0.15–0.3 ml/kg/hr as 50% ethanol in fruit juice.

17. Morphine, Heroin

Naloxone: 0.1 mg/kg/dose IV. Maximum 2 mg.

18. Organophosphorus

- Atropine: 0.05 mg/kg IV, repeat q5–10 min till atropinization occurs, then repeat the dose q30–60 min or give IV infusion 0.02–0.08 mg/kg/hr.
- Pralidoxine 2-pyridime aldozime methiodide (PAM): 25–50 mg/kg diluted in 5% NS and given over 5–30 min. May be repeated after 1 hr and repeat doses q6–12 hr.
- Severe poisoning IV infusion rate is 9–19 mg/kg/hr.

19. Phenothiazine

Diphenhydramine: 1–3 mg/kg IV q30 min, may be repeated after 3–4 hr IM/oral (maximum dose: 300 mg/day).

20. Scorpion bite

Prazocin: 0.25 mg oral q4–6 hr for 24 hr

21. Methemoglobinemia

Methylene blue: 1–2 mg/kg IV 1% solution over 5–10 minutes. Maximum dose: 7 mg/kg.

22. Digitalis toxicity

- Digoxin immune Fab antibody (Digiband)
- Depends on body load of digoxin, determined as milligrams of digoxin ingested × 0.8.
- 1 vial (40 mg) dissolved in 4 ml sterile water given over 30 minutes.

23. Sulphonylurea

Octreotide: 1 µg/kg/dose q12 hr

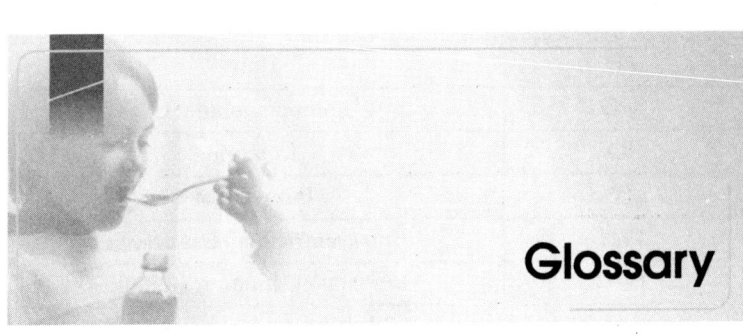

Glossary

ABC	Airway, breathing, circulation
ABG	Arterial blood gases
ACTH	Adrenocorticotropic hormone
ADE	Adverse drug effects
ADR	Adverse drug reactions
AED	Antiepileptic drug
AEFI	Adverse effects following immunisation
ATT	Antituberculous therapy
BD	Twice a day
BMI	Body mass index
BP	Blood pressure
BUN	Blood urea nitrogen
BW	Body weight
CCF	Congestive cardiac failure
Cap	Capsule
CSF	Cerebrospinal fluid
DIC	Disseminated intravascular coagulopathy
Div	Divided
ET	Endotracheal
Hib	*Haemophillus influenzae b*
HIV	Human immunodeficiency virus

Hr	Hour
IgG	Immunoglobulin G
IO	Intraoral
IV	Intravenous
IVH	Intraventricular hemorrhage
IVIG	Intravenous immunoglobulins
MDR strains	Multidrug resistant strains
Min	Minutes
MMR	Measles-mumps-rubella
MRSA	Methicillin resistant *Staphylococcus aureus*
NG	Nasogastric
PEM	Protein energy malnutrition
O	Orally
PDA	Patent ductus arteriosis
PO	Per oral
PR	Per rectum
q	Every
ROP	Retinopathy of prematurity
SAM	Severe acute malnutrition
SC	Subcutaneous
Sec	Seconds
Susp	Suspension
Syr	Syrup
Tabs	Tablets
TDS	Three times a day
VRSA	Vancomysin resistant *Staphylococcus aureus*
Wk	Week
Wt	Weight
Yr	Year

Measurements

Imperial	Metric
1/4 tsp	1 ml
1/2 tsp	2 ml
1 tsp	5 ml
1 tbsp	15 ml
1/4 cup	50 ml
1/3 cup	75 ml
1/2 cup	125 ml
2/3 cup	150 ml
3/4 cup	175 ml
1 cup	250 ml
1 pint	500 ml
1 quart	1 liter

Liquid Measurements

1/2 fl oz	15 ml	1 tbsp
1 fl oz	30 ml	1/8 cup
2 fl oz	60 ml	1/4 cup
4 fl oz	120 ml	1/2 cup
8 fl oz	240 ml	1 cup
16 fl oz	480 ml	1 pint

Liquid Equivalents

2 cups	1 pint	1/2 quart
4 cups	2 pints	1 quart
4 pints	2 quarts	1/2 gallon
8 pints	4 quarts	1 gallon

Weights	
Imperial	*Metric*
1 ounce	28 grams
2 ounces	55 grams
3 ounces	85 grams
4 ounces	115 grams
8 ounces	225 grams
16 ounces	455 grams

Temperatures			
Fahrenheit	*Celsius*	*Gas Mark*	*Description*
32	0		
212	100		
250	120	1/2	
275	140	1	Cool
300	150	2	
325	160	3	Very moderate
350	180	4	Moderate
375	190	5	
400	200	6	Moderately hot
425	220	7	Hot
450	230	8	
475	240	9	Very hot
500	260		

Index